617.75

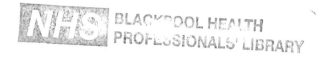
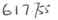
The Blackpool, Fylde & Wyre
Health Library

This book is due for return on or before the last date shown below
to avoid overdue charges.
Books may be renewed (twice only) unless required by other readers.
Renewals may be made in person or by telephone, quoting reader number
and the number on the barcode below.

Clinical Management of Myopia

Clinical Management of Myopia

Theodore Grosvenor, O.D., Ph.D., F.A.A.O.
Professor Emeritus, School of Optometry,
Indiana University, Bloomington;
Visiting Scholar, Department of Optometry and Vision Science,
University of Auckland, Auckland, New Zealand

David A. Goss, O.D., Ph.D., F.A.A.O.
Professor, School of Optometry,
Indiana University, Bloomington

With a Foreword by
Henry W Hofstetter, O.D, Ph.D., F.A.A.O.
Rudy Professor Emeritus of Optometry,
School of Optometry,
Indiana University, Bloomington

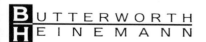

BUTTERWORTH
HEINEMANN

Boston   Oxford   Auckland   Johannesburg   Melbourne   New Delhi

Every effort has been made to ensure that the drug dosage schedules within this text are accurate and conform to standards accepted at time of publication. However, as treatment recommendations vary in the light of continuing research and clinical experience, the reader is advised to verify drug dosage schedules herein with information found on product information sheets. This is especially true in cases of new or infrequently used drugs.

∞ Recognizing the importance of preserving what has been written, Butter-worth–Heinemann prints its books on acid-free paper whenever possible.

 Butterworth–Heinemann supports the efforts of American Forests and the Global ReLeaf program in its campaign for the betterment of trees, forests, and our environment.

Library of Congress Cataloging-in-Publication Data

Grosvenor, Theodore P.
    Clinical management of myopia / Theodore Grosvenor, David A. Goss;
    foreword by Henry W. Hofstetter.
        p.   cm.
    Includes bibliographical references and index.
    ISBN 0-7506-7060-6
    1. Myopia. I. Goss, David A., 1948- . II. Title
    [DNLM: 1. Myopia--epidemiology. 2. Myopia--diagnosis. 3. Myopia-
-surgery. 4. Optometry--methods. WW 320 G879c 1999]
RE938.G67 1999
617.7'55--dc21
DNLM/DLC
for Library of Congress   98-46246
                          CIP

British Library Cataloguing-in-Publication Data
A catalogue record for this book is available from the British Library.

The publisher offers special discounts on bulk orders of this book.
For information, please contact:

Manager of Special Sales
Butterworth–Heinemann
225 Wildwood Avenue
Woburn, MA 01801-2041
Tel: 781-904-2500
Fax: 781-904-2620

For information on all Butterworth–Heinemann publications available, contact our World Wide Web home page at: http://www.bh.com

10 9 8 7 6 5 4 3 2 1

Printed in the United States of America

To our wives, Betty and Dawn,
for their understanding and encouragement

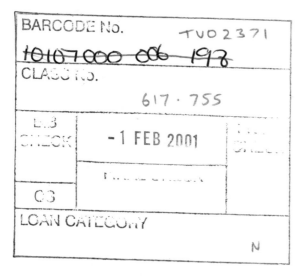

Near-sightedness is usually the result of occupation or habits requiring the close and minute examination of small objects.
—Herman von Helmholtz (1866)

The traditional emphasis on environmental factors as productive of refractive errors finds no support in the detailed studies of today.
—Arnold Sorsby (1966)

Science has been likened to a soccer game played by eight-year-olds. They all kick the ball around here until someone kicks it out over there; then they all run out and kick the ball around over there.
—William H. Miller (1990)

Evidence is strong that both genetics and environment are potential determinants of myopia.
—Wendy Marsh-Tootle (1998)

Because appreciable differences in refractive error result from very slight anatomical deviations, it is likely that much variation in refractive error may be unattributable to particular genetic or environmental influences, no matter how well these come to be measured and characterized.
—John C. Bear (1991)

Education's purpose is to replace an empty mind with an open one.
—Malcolm S. Forbes (1983)

The characteristics of a good clinician can be represented by four Cs: competency, compassion, curiosity, and common sense.
—Paraphrased from C. Everett Koop

Concerning the age-related shift toward hyperopia in late adulthood: I was slightly myopic most of my adult life and I enjoyed it. The ability to shave and read without specs was a real advantage, which I now miss, being essentially emmetropic. . . . I think that there are going to be a number of very unhappy senior citizens who had successful refractive surgery when young adults.
—Meredith W. Morgan (1991)

Contents

Foreword   xi
Henry W Hofstetter
Preface   xiii

I. GENERAL PRINCIPLES

1. Epidemiology of Myopia   3
Optics of the Myopic Eye   3
Prevalence of Myopia   8
Classification of Myopia   14
Risk Factors for Myopia Onset   16
Progression of Myopia   21
Pathologic Changes in Myopia   31
Ocular Morbidity Due to Myopia   39

2. Etiology of Myopia   49
Is Myopia the Result of Inheritance, Environmental
    Factors, or Both?   49
Can We Identify Likely Physiologic Mechanisms by Which
    Near Work Plays a Role in Myopia Development?   51
Given the Likely Physiologic Mechanisms of Near
    Work–Induced Myopia, Can We Identify Potential
    Methods of Myopia Control or Prevention?   58
Conclusion   58

3. Clinical Examination   63
Symptoms of Myopia   63
Refractive Examination   68
Binocular Vision Examination   70
Ocular Health Examination   74

4. Prescribing for Myopia   77
General Guidelines   77
Accommodation and Vergence Considerations   79
Presbyopia   84
Glasses or Contact Lenses?   86
Spectacle Lens Considerations   91
Night Myopia and Pseudomyopia   92
Induced Myopia   94
Conclusion and Comments   95

II. METHODS OF MYOPIA CONTROL AND REDUCTION

5. **Vision Therapy**   **101**
   The Baltimore Project   101
   Biofeedback Studies   102
   Studies on Various Behavioral Training Methods   105
   Vision Therapy Programs for Myopia Control   107
   Conclusion and Comments   109

6. **Control with Added Plus Power for Near Work**   **113**
   Bifocals   113
   Progressive Addition Lenses   125
   Undercorrection   125
   Part-Time Wear of Spectacles   125
   Summary of Study Results   126
   Power to Use in Bifocals   126
   Comments on Patient Education   126

7. **Myopia Control with Pharmaceutical Agents**   **129**
   Cycloplegic Agents   129
   Adrenergic Blocking Agents   134
   Future Possibilities: Agents Acting on the Retina   134

8. **Corneal Topography Measurement**   **139**
   Peripheral Keratometry   139
   Photokeratoscopy   144
   Videokeratoscopy   144

9. **Myopia Control or Reduction with Rigid Contact Lenses**   **155**
   Control of Progression with Conventionally Fitted
      Rigid Lenses   155
   Orthokeratology with Conventionally Designed Rigid Lenses   163
   Accelerated Orthokeratology with Reverse Geometry Lenses   167
   Orthokeratology after Refractive Surgery   177

10. **Keratorefractive Surgery**   **181**
    Radial Keratotomy   181
    Laser Photorefractive Keratectomy   187
    Automated Lamellar Keratoplasty   197
    Laser in situ Keratomileusis   198
    Intrastromal Corneal Ring   200
    Comanagement of Refractive Surgery Patients   201

11. **Refractive Surgery Involving the Lens**   **207**
    Clear Lens Extraction   207
    Intraocular Lens Implantation in a Phakic Eye   211

    Index   **219**

Foreword

The invitation to write a foreword to this text reminded me momentarily of a professional adage I heard long ago as a teenaged freshman chemistry student at Adelbert College of Western Reserve University. It had to do with the significance of the difference between fiddle-dee-dee and fiddle-dee-dum in scientific research.

At that time, the word *myopia* was not in my vocabulary, and if I was already myopic, I was unaware of it for at least another 2 years. On eventually being informed that I was "nearsighted," I interpreted this merely as a distance differentiation from farsightedness not unlike the fiddle-dee-dee and fiddle-dee-dum distinction. Far and near were merely two points on a continuous linear scale.

The oneness of the range of ocular refraction was further reinforced later in my first year of the optometry curriculum at The Ohio State University. Southall's derivation of a single, thin lens formula for all powers in his geometric optics text crystallized the concept. It was not until I was enrolled in clinical courses and actually prescribing lenses that I discovered a strange caution on the part of several of my supervisors who were privately practicing optometrists. They were quite consistently unwilling to approve an overcorrection, or even a full correction, of minus lenses, but showed no hesitation to approve an undercorrection of hyperopia. They defended their advice as the result of "clinical experience." My perusal of the optometric literature showed a dearth of statistical evidence to support their advice, but the anecdotally established opinion among practicing optometrists seemed ubiquitous.

A little later in my career I happened to gain access to the files of a practicing optometrist of advanced years whose records included many repeat patients. I used the opportunity to undertake a statistical study of the interrelationship of age, refraction, and rates of refractive change.* The plotted data clearly suggested that myopia and hyperopia were different in their development. Hyperopia tended to be static, whereas myopia seemed to beget myopia. Fiddle-dee-dee did indeed differ from fiddle-dee-dum.

The authors of this book are well matched to explore the clinical management of myopia as a uniquely identifiable functional entity. Drs. Grosvenor and Goss come from very different academic backgrounds,

---

*Am J Optom Arch Am Acad Optom 1954;31:161–169.

philosophically, and significantly different generations. Their coming together at Indiana University was pure happenstance a few short years ago. They soon realized that their efforts and interests were highly complementary. They are quite aware that the concepts of myopia that evolved during the decades of my own career reflect many parallels in the clinical profession at large and have tailored the book accordingly. It may well be the optometric contribution of the year.

HENRY W HOFSTETTER

Preface

Myopia is both the easiest and one of the most difficult problems a vision care practitioner must treat. It is the easiest problem because prescribing minus lenses for healthy, previously uncorrected myopic eyes will undoubtedly improve visual acuity and thus eliminate symptoms of blurred distance vision. It is one of the most difficult problems because the practitioner may not be sure that the chosen method of correction is the best for the patient or whether other forms of management may be likely to reduce the rate of progression. And when compared with emmetropic, hyperopic, or astigmatic eyes, myopic eyes are known to be at greater risk for retinal detachment, chorioretinal degeneration, and glaucoma.

Should glasses that provide the best distance visual acuity be prescribed for constant wear? Should conventional vision therapy or biofeedback training for myopia reduction be undertaken? Should a plus add be prescribed to reduce the demand on accommodation for near work? If so, should the add be in the form of reading glasses, bifocals, or progressive addition lenses? And should a plus add be considered only on the basis of the refractive error, or should the patient's binocular vision status be taken into consideration?

Should conventional rigid contact lenses be prescribed to reduce the rate of progression of juvenile myopia? Should orthokeratology be undertaken, with the goal of reducing the existing amount of myopia? Should an atropine-like agent be prescribed for daily use? Should keratorefractive surgery be considered, and if so, which of the alphabet soup of procedures—RK, PRK, ALK, LASIK, or others yet to be developed?

During the past few decades, the results of retrospective and prospective clinical studies of all of these methods of myopia management have appeared in the vision care literature. This text reviews and evaluates these studies, providing practitioners, teachers, and students of optometry with the latest and most thorough information on the clinical management of myopia. Also included is information on the nature and etiology of myopia and clinical examination methods, to serve as a background for the discussions of myopia management.

The intent of this book is not to present an all-inclusive review of all publications on myopia but to provide comprehensive coverage of key studies that have implications for clinical management of myopia. Neither is it the goal of this book to give unconditional answers to the questions posed above but rather to equip the reader with the knowledge to approach those questions when presented with the unique complex of needs, expectations, demographic characteristics, and clinical findings each patient offers.

In categorizing methods of managing myopia, we have used the terms *myopia correction*, *myopia control*, and *myopia reduction*. *Myopia correction* refers to the prescription of spectacle lenses or contact lenses to provide clear, comfortable, efficient vision. A semantic purist might suggest that we should substitute the term *myopia compensation* because we are actually optically compensating for the myopia rather than actually correcting the disorder. However, discussions of "correcting" refractive errors seem to be ingrained in the jargon, so we have retained the use of the term *myopia correction*. *Myopia control* refers to clinical regimens designed to control the rate of myopia progression; *myopia reduction* refers to methods of reducing or eliminating myopia. It should be understood that none of the methods of myopia control or reduction currently available can provide guaranteed results. We have endeavored to provide, for all methods of myopia control or reduction, sufficient background information, including the results of clinical studies, to enable the practitioner to make a judgment concerning the use of a specific method for a specific patient. If myopia could be successfully managed by "cookbook" methods, what need would there be for the vision care professions?

We thank Dr. Rodger Kame for suggesting that this book be written and the staff at Butterworth–Heinemann for their confidence in us and their support: Barbara Murphy for initiating the project and Karen Oberheim and Leslie Kramer for seeing it to completion. We also thank Terri Greene, faculty secretary at Indiana University School of Optometry, for her assistance.

THEODORE GROSVENOR
DAVID A. GOSS

Clinical
Management
of Myopia

PART **I**

General Principles

CHAPTER 1

Epidemiology of Myopia

Patients with myopia can see near objects clearly, but distant objects are blurred. Thus, a behavioral definition of myopia could be an inability to see well in the distance without optical correction, while good near vision is retained. An optical definition of myopia is a refractive condition in which parallel rays are focused in front of the retina with accommodation at a zero level. The clinical management of myopia can consist of (1) *myopia correction*, optical compensation for the myopia with minus lenses to improve distance visual acuity; (2) *myopia control*, techniques for slowing the rate of myopia progression; and/or (3) *myopia reduction*, techniques to reduce the amount of an existing myopia.

Myopia is a very common condition, and it has been studied extensively. The etiology of myopia is not well understood, but the descriptive characteristics of myopia are well known. A knowledge of these descriptive characteristics is helpful in trying to understand the etiology of myopia, in making informed lens prescribing decisions, in designing appropriate myopia control and myopia reduction techniques, and in communicating effectively with patients and other professionals. This chapter touches on the optics of the myopic eye, the prevalence of myopia, the natural history of myopia, risk factors for myopia development, the sequelae of myopia, and related topics.

Optics of the Myopic Eye

Focus of parallel rays of light (light from infinity) in front of the retina could occur by having a vitreous depth that is *too great for the refractive power* of the eye or an ocular refractive power that is *too great for the vitreous depth* of the eye. The optics of the myopic eye can be examined in two ways: (1) by comparison studies, in which ocular optical component data are compared in myopes and nonmyopes, and (2) by correlation studies, in which coefficients of correlation of refractive error with the various ocular optical components have been calculated.

Correlation Studies

The results of seven studies that presented correlations of refractive error with axial length, corneal power, and crystalline lens power are summarized in Table 1.1. The highest correlations are those of refractive error with axial length and with vitreous depth. The negative sign indicates a more minus refractive error is correlated with a greater axial length or a greater vitreous depth.

The correlation of refractive error with corneal power is negative, indicating an association of more minus refractive error with greater corneal power. This correlation is lower in magnitude than that of refractive error and axial length. To determine whether the correlation of refractive error and corneal power was low in part because it was overwhelmed by the strong correlation of refractive error and axial length, two studies calculated partial correlation coefficients. Using Stenstrom's data, van Alphen (1961) found that the correlation of refractive error with corneal power increased from –0.18 to –0.67 when axial length was factored out. Similarly, Goss et al. (1997) noted that the correlation of refractive error with anterior corneal radius of curvature increased from 0.28 to 0.62 when the effect of vitreous depth was factored out.

The coefficients of correlation of refractive error with crystalline lens power were very low and usually positive. A positive correlation indicates an association of more myopic refractive error with lesser crystalline lens powers. This suggests that the crystalline lens does not contribute to myopia because lesser refractive powers would produce a tendency toward hyperopia. Thus, these correlation studies suggest that myopia is associated mainly with a greater axial length and, to a lesser extent, is related to greater corneal powers.

Comparison Studies

Numerous studies have shown axial length or vitreous depth to be greater in myopic eyes than in emmetropic eyes. For example, Curtin (1985) cited measurements reported by Tron in 1929 in which axial lengths ranged from 20.5 to 25.5 mm in emmetropia, from 21.6 to 26.4 mm in low myopia (up to –6 D), and from 21.9 to 34.8 mm in high myopia (greater than –6 D). Sorsby et al. (1962) reported that the axial length of 107 emmetropic eyes (refractive errors 0.00 to +0.50 D) ranged from 22.3 to 26.0 mm. Of 37 eyes with myopia greater than –4.0 D, the shortest axial length was 25.8 mm, and 34 of 37 eyes had axial lengths greater than 26.0 mm. Data collected from clinical microscopists in Great Britain by McBrien and Adams (1997) are summarized in Table 1.2. Vitreous depths were greater in both youth-onset myopes and early adult–onset myopes than in emmetropes. Ocular optical component data for emmetropic and myopic Oklahoma optometry students are compared in Tables 1.3–1.5. Because males tend to have larger eyes with flatter corneas, males and females were considered separately.

TABLE 1.1
Coefficients of Correlation (r) of Refractive Error with the Optical Components:
Data from Seven Studies

Study	Study Sample	Axial Length	Power of Anterior Corneal Surface	Crystalline Lens Power
Stenstrom (1948a,b)	n = 1,000 20–35 yrs old Sweden	–0.76	–0.18	0.00
Ohno (1956)	n = 495 14–16 yrs old Japan	–0.60	–0.11	+0.39
van Alphen (1961)[a]	n = 194 ≤50 yrs old Great Britain	–0.77	–0.30	+0.28
Araki (1962)	n = 295 9–56 yrs old Japan	–0.77	–0.17	+0.02
Garner et al. (1990)	n = 904 7–17 yrs old Malaysia	–0.77	–0.12	+0.30
Goss et al. (1990)	n = 1,286 6–40 yrs old Several data sources	Males: –0.74 Females: –0.76	Males: –0.14 Females: –0.07	—
Goss et al. (1997)	n = 176 20–44 yrs old Oklahoma	–0.71[b]	–0.28	+0.08

[a]Using data of Sorsby et al. (1957).
[b]Correlation of refractive error with vitreous depth.

Vitreous depth averaged 16.85 mm in female myopes compared with 15.83 mm in female emmetropes, and 17.13 mm in male myopes compared with 16.33 mm in male emmetropes. Vitreous depth was significantly greater in subjects with myopia than in those with emmetropia.

Curtin (1985) noted that studies by Schiotz, Valk, Sulzer, and Steiger in the late nineteenth and early twentieth centuries reported corneal powers to be greater in myopes than in emmetropes and hyperopes. Curtin stated that

TABLE 1.2
Ocular Optical Component Data for Subjects between 21 and 61 Years of Age

	Emmetropia	Youth-Onset Myopia	Adult-Onset Myopia
Number of subjects	68	47	78
Refractive error			
Mean	+0.10	–3.74	–1.68
SE	0.03	0.31	0.13
Corneal radius (mm)			
Mean	7.89	7.85	7.85
SE	0.03	0.05	0.03
Anterior chamber depth (mm)			
Mean	3.51	3.76	3.69
SE	0.04	0.07	0.05
Crystalline lens thickness (mm)			
Mean	3.96	3.91	3.88
SE	0.05	0.07	0.05
Vitreous depth (mm)			
Mean	16.23	17.80	17.14
SE	0.08	0.16	0.12
Axial length			
Mean	23.69	25.47	24.71
SE	0.08	0.17	0.12

SE = standard error.
Source: Data from NA McBrien, DW Adams. A longitudinal investigation of adult-onset and adult-progression of myopia in an occupational group—refractive and biometric findings. Invest Ophthalmol Vis Sci 1997;38:321–333.

Steiger found mean corneal power to be approximately 43.63 D in both emmetropic and hyperopic eyes, but almost 1 D greater in myopic eyes. Sorsby et al. (1957) gave mean corneal powers of 43.25 D for 90 emmetropic eyes and 44.40 D for 42 myopic eyes. In three studies comparing ocular optical components in subjects who had onset of myopia in early adulthood (and had fairly low amounts of myopia) with subjects who were emmetropic, McBrien and Millodot (1987) and Bullimore et al. (1992) did not find a significant difference in corneal powers, but Grosvenor and Scott (1991) found mean corneal power to be 1.12 D greater in the myopes ($p < .01$). The data of McBrien and Adams (1997) given in Table 1.2 show a tendency of steeper corneas in myopia than in emmetropia, but the difference was not statistically significant.

Scott and Grosvenor (1993) compared corneal radius in 42 emmetropic adults (refractive errors of –0.50 to +1.50 D) to those of 42 myopic adults (–5.00 to –7.00 D). The mean corneal radius was 7.83 mm in the emmetropes and 7.70 mm in the myopes. The data of Goss et al. (1997) in Tables 1.3–1.5 show significantly steeper corneas in myopes than in emmetropes. Overall, then, most studies find mean corneal powers to be greater in myopia than in

TABLE 1.3
Ocular Components in Emmetropic and Myopic Female Optometry
Students in Oklahoma

	Emmetropes			*Myopes*		
	n	*Mean*	*SD*	*n*	*Mean*	*SD*
Anterior chamber depth (mm)	19	3.72	0.32	44	3.80	0.28
Crystalline lens thickness (mm)	19	3.69	0.31	44	3.66	0.23
Vitreous depth (mm)	19	15.83	0.64	44	16.85	0.77
Vertical corneal radius (mm)	19	7.60	0.22	44	7.57	0.20
Anterior lens radius (mm)	18	9.57	0.94	37	9.78	1.11
Posterior lens radius (mm)	18	−5.68	0.50	37	−5.83	0.57
Crystalline lens power (D)	18	21.48	1.50	37	20.56	2.45
Vertical meridian retinoscopy (D)	19	+0.17	0.36	44	−3.42	2.20

Source: Reprinted with permission from DA Goss, HG VanVeen, BB Rainey, B Feng. Ocular components measured by keratometry, phakometry, and ultrasonography in emmetropic and myopic optometry students. Optom Vis Sci 1997;74:489–495.

emmetropia. It should be noted, however, that there is considerable variability in corneal power in both emmetropia and myopia. For example, Sorsby et al. (1962) reported corneal power ranged from 39.0 to 47.6 D in 107 emmetropic eyes.

Using comparison phakometry, Sheridan (1955) found no significant difference in anterior crystalline lens radius between emmetropic eyes and myopic eyes of adults. Garner et al. (1992) calculated crystalline lens power from other optical components in Malay children ranging in age from 9 to 15 years. The mean crystalline lens power for 19 emmetropes (mean refractive error, +0.01 D) was 22.88 D, with a standard deviation of 1.66 D. The average crystalline lens power for 19 myopes (mean refractive error, −6.08 D) was 20.58 D, with a standard deviation of 2.14 D. The difference was statistically significant ($p < .05$). The data of Goss at al. (1997) in Tables 1.3–1.5 do not show a statistically significant difference in crystalline lens power between emmetropes and myopes, but they do show a slight trend toward flatter posterior lens surface curvature in myopes, which is consistent with the lower crystalline lens power in myopes found by Garner et al.

TABLE 1.4
Ocular Components in Emmetropic and Myopic Male Optometry
Students in Oklahoma

	Emmetropes			Myopes		
	n	Mean	SD	n	Mean	SD
Anterior chamber depth (mm)	34	3.86	0.28	71	3.92	0.31
Crystalline lens thickness (mm)	34	3.63	0.25	71	3.62	0.24
Vitreous depth (mm)	34	16.33	0.62	71	17.13	0.94
Vertical corneal radius (mm)	34	7.77	0.26	71	7.63	0.22
Anterior lens radius (mm)	32	10.05	0.86	66	9.88	1.16
Posterior lens radius (mm)	32	–5.93	0.43	66	–6.10	0.59
Crystalline lens power (D)	32	20.35	1.07	66	20.39	1.69
Vertical meridian retinoscopy (D)	34	+0.25	0.36	71	–2.87	2.14

Source: Reprinted with permission from DA Goss, HG VanVeen, BB Rainey, B Feng. Ocular components measured by keratometry, phakometry, and ultrasonography in emmetropic and myopic optometry students. Optom Vis Sci 1997;74:489–495.

Summary of Optics of the Myopic Eye

Both the correlation and the comparison studies show that the myopic eye is a long eye due to enlargement of the vitreous chamber. The myopic eye also tends to have a steeper cornea, although there is considerable variability in corneal power in both emmetropes and myopes. There may also be a tendency toward lesser crystalline lens power in myopia, perhaps due to a slightly flatter posterior surface. Some studies have found greater anterior chamber depths in myopes than in emmetropes (Curtin, 1985; Grosvenor, 1994; McBrien and Adams, 1997), but the magnitude of the difference suggests that it contributes little to the dioptric difference in refractive error (Erickson, 1977, 1984, 1991; Goss and Erickson, 1990). The dioptric difference in refractive error between myopic and emmetropic eyes is primarily due to *greater vitreous depth* in myopic eyes and secondarily to greater corneal power.

Prevalence of Myopia

Many factors affect the prevalence of myopia. A major factor is age. Prevalences of myopia at different ages as found in various studies are summarized in Tables 1.6–1.9. Other factors affecting myopia prevalence include

TABLE 1.5

Statistical Significance (*p* Values) of Difference in Ocular Components between Emmetropes and Myopes and between Males and Females Tested by Analysis of Variance

	Refractive Group	Gender
Anterior chamber depth	0.197	0.010
Crystalline lens thickness	0.695	0.213
Vitreous depth	<0.001	0.008
Vertical corneal radius	0.008	0.009
Anterior lens radius	0.854	0.212
Posterior lens radius	0.086	0.005
Crystalline lens power	0.315	0.111

Source: Reprinted with permission from DA Goss, HG VanVeen, BB Rainey, B Feng. Ocular components measured by keratometry, phakometry, and ultrasonography in emmetropic and myopic optometry students. Optom Vis Sci 1997;74:489–495.

educational attainment, occupation, amount of reading and near work, gender, socioeconomic status, and ethnic heritage.

Prevalence Among Newborns and Preschool Children

The prevalence of myopia among newborns is high, approximately 25% in two studies (Cook and Glasscock, 1951; Goldschmidt, 1969) and 50% in another (Mohindra and Held, 1981). Myopia is very common among premature (low-birth-weight) infants, although it usually reduces to emmetropia by 1 year of age (Fletcher and Brandon, 1955; Scharf et al., 1975; Yamamoto et al., 1979). The myopia of low-birth-weight infants is thought to be largely due to the steep corneas of their immature eyes (Fledelius, 1981; Goss, 1985).

Both myopia and hyperopia decrease in amount over the first few years of life, with most of the change occurring in the first year (Ingram and Barr, 1979; Mohindra and Held, 1981; Ehrlich et al., 1997). This shift in refractive error toward emmetropia is referred to as *emmetropization*. As the eye grows, vitreous depth increases, which by itself would cause a shift toward myopia, and the refractive powers of the cornea and crystalline lens decrease, which by themselves would cause a shift toward hyperopia. Emmetropization can be explained by a counterbalancing of these changes, as a coarse control mechanism, along with modulation of axial elongation of the eye by feedback from retinal image clarity, as a fine control mechanism (Goss and Wickham, 1995; Grosvenor, 1996). At approximately 5 or 6 years of age, when children start school, myopia prevalence is at the lowest of any time during the human life span—approximately 1% or 2%—as noted in Table 1.6.

Prevalence of Myopia in School-Age Children

Many children who enter school as emmetropes become myopic during the school-age years. Prevalences of myopia for school-age children from vari-

TABLE 1.6
Prevalence of Myopia for Children from Birth to Ages 6–8,
from Various Studies Compiled by Grosvenor

Age (years)	Source	Subject	Criterion	Prevalence (%)
Birth	Cook and Glasscock (1951)	Caucasian	Any myopia	24
Birth	Goldschmidt (1969)	Danish	Any myopia	25
Birth	Mohindra and Held (1981)	Boston area	Any myopia	50
5–6	Hirsch (1952)	Los Angeles	–1.00 D or more	1
6	Blum et al. (1959)	Orinda, CA	–0.50 D or more	2
6	Hirsch (1964)	Ojai, CA	–0.50 D or more	2
6–8	Kempf et al. (1928)	Caucasian	Any myopia	2
7–8	Laatikainen and Erkkila (1980)	Finnish	–0.50 D or more	2
7	Mäntyjärvi (1983)	Finnish	–0.25 D or more	1

Source: Reprinted with permission from T Grosvenor. A review and a suggested classification system for myopia on the basis of age-related prevalence and age of onset. Am J Optom Physiol Opt 1987;64:545–554.

TABLE 1.7
Prevalence of Myopia during the School Years, from Various Studies
Compiled by Grosvenor

Age (years)	Source	Subject	Criterion	Prevalence (%)
6–11	U.S. Department of Health, Education, and Welfare (1978)	NPS[a]	Wearing a correction[b]	6
13–14	Hirsch (1952)	Los Angeles	–1.00 D or more	5
13–14	Hirsch (1952)	Los Angeles	–0.25 D or more	23
14	Blum et al. (1959)	Orinda, CA	–0.50 D or more	15
14	Hirsch (1964)	Ojai, CA	–0.50 D or more	12
14–15	Laatikainen and Erkkila (1980)	Finnish	–0.50 D or more	22
15	Mäntyjärvi (1983)	Finnish	–0.25 D or more	23
12–17	U.S. Dept. of Health, Education, and Welfare (1978)	NPS[a]	Wearing a correction	26

[a]National probability sample of U.S. population ages 4–74 years.
[b]Currently wearing a correction (glasses or contact lenses) for myopia.
Source: Reprinted with permission from T Grosvenor. A review and a suggested classification system for myopia on the basis of age-related prevalence and age of onset. Am J Optom Physiol Opt 1987;64:545–554.

TABLE 1.8
Prevalence of Myopia during the Early Adult Years,
from Various Studies Compiled by Grosvenor

Age (years)	Source	Subject	Criterion	Prevalence (%)
18–24	U.S. Dept. of Health, Education, and Welfare (1978)	NPS[a]	Wearing a correction[b]	33
20–30	Borish (1970)	Jackson (1932) and Tassman (1932) data	>–0.50 D	22
25–34	U.S. Dept. of Health, Education, and Welfare (1978)	NPS[a]	Wearing a correction[b]	34
26–35	Fledelius (1983)	Hospital patients	–0.25 D or more	41
30–40	Borish (1970)	Jackson (1932) and Tassman (1932) data	>–0.50 D	16
35–44	U.S. Dept. of Health, Education, and Welfare (1978)	NPS[a]	Wearing a correction[b]	31
36–45	Fledelius (1983)	Hospital patients	–0.25 D or more	33

[a]National probability sample of U.S. population ages 4–74 years.
[b]Currently wearing a correction (glasses or contact lenses) for myopia.
Source: Reprinted with permission from T Grosvenor. A review and a suggested classification system for myopia on the basis of age-related prevalence and age of onset. Am J Optom Physiol Opt 1987;64:545–554.

ous studies are summarized in Tables 1.7 and 1.10. Although the data in Table 1.10 are now somewhat old, they suggest that the most common time of myopia onset is around 9–12 years of age and its onset in girls may precede that in boys by a year or two. Richler and Bear (1980) also noted that a tendency toward earlier onset in girls than in boys. In the United States and Western countries, the prevalence of myopia in children ages 5–6 years is 1–2%, and the prevalence in the late teens is approximately 25%.

Prevalence in the Early Adult Years

The results of some studies giving prevalence for young adults are summarized in Table 1.8. It appears that the prevalence of myopia among young

TABLE 1.9
Prevalence of Myopia during the Later Adult Years,
from Various Studies Compiled by Grosvenor

Age (years)	Source	Subject	Criterion	Prevalence (%)
45–49	Hirsch (1958)	Optometric patients	–1.13 D or more	7
40–50	Borish (1970)	Jackson (1932) and Tassman (1932) data	>–0.50 D	14
45–54	U.S. Dept. of Health, Education, and Welfare (1978)	NPS[a]	Wearing a correction[b]	32
46–55	Fledelius (1983)	Hospital patients	–0.25 D or more	26
55–64	U.S. Dept. of Health, Education, and Welfare (1978)	NPS[a]	Wearing a correction[b]	18
56–65	Fledelius (1983)	Hospital patients	–0.25 D or more	26
65–74	U.S. Dept. of Health, Education, and Welfare (1978)	NPS[a]	Wearing a correction[b]	16
>66	Fledelius (1983)	Hospital patients	–0.25 D or more	14
>70	Borish (1970)	Jackson (1932) and Tassman (1932) data	>–0.50 D	21
>75	Hirsch (1958)	Optometric patients	–1.13 D or more	15

[a]National probability sample of U.S. population ages 4–74 years.
[b]Currently wearing a correction (glasses or contact lenses) for myopia.
Source: Reprinted with permission from T Grosvenor. A review and a suggested classification system for myopia on the basis of age-related prevalence and age of onset. Am J Optom Physiol Opt 1987;64:545–554.

adults in the United States and Western countries reaches approximately 30–35% by about 40 years of age.

Prevalence in the Later Adult Years

Prevalence data for the later adult years are given in Table 1.9. Many patients with myopia experience decreases after age 45 years, and some shift from myopia back into hyperopia. The result is that the prevalence of

TABLE 1.10
Prevalence of Myopia among Schoolchildren in the Los Angeles Area
and Pullman, Washington

	Hirsch (1952)				*Young et al. (1954)*	
	Children with Myopia of Any Amount (%)		*Children with Myopia >1 D (%)*		*Children with Myopia >1 D (%)*	
Age (years)	*Girls*	*Boys*	*Girls*	*Boys*	*Girls*	*Boys*
5–6	6.15	7.43	0.45	0.67	4.17	0.00
7–8	9.71	11.02	0.98	0.90	2.60	5.62
9–10	17.18	15.68	2.01	1.82	19.44	9.68
11–12	21.60	20.74	5.77	3.08	20.00	27.27
13–14	25.36	22.53	5.78	5.08	25.71	28.57

Sources: Data from MJ Hirsch. The changes in refraction between the ages of 5 and 14—theoretical and practical considerations. Am J Optom Arch Am Acad Optom 1952;29:445–459; and FA Young, RJ Beattie, FJ Newby, MT Swindal. The Pullman study—a visual survey of Pullman schoolchildren. Part II. Am J Optom Arch Am Acad Optom 1954;31:192–203.

myopia for patients older than age 45 years is lower than it is at age 30–40 years, when prevalence peaks at 30–35%. Hirsch (1958) reported refractive data for patients in the later adult years from his private practice in California. Because almost all persons with presbyopia seek clinical care, clinical data may be a "less selected" sample at those ages than at other times in the life span. Hirsch found the median refractive error of his patients to increase from +0.18 D at 45–49 years to +1.02 D at age 75 years and older. However, he noted that in some patients refractive error shifted in the direction of myopia as a result of age-related nuclear cataracts. This can result in onset of myopia in some persons approximately 60 years of age and older, and may be the most common cause of late adult–onset myopia.

Other Factors Related to Prevalence

In a study in the United States, Sperduto et al. (1983) found a higher prevalence of myopia for females than for males, and a higher prevalence among whites than among black Americans. The prevalence of myopia was higher for higher family income levels and for more years of schooling. Angle and Wissman (1980) found that the prevalence of myopia for Americans ages 12–17 years was higher in females than in males and higher in whites than in black Americans. They also found that greater prevalence was associated with higher income, greater daily reading time, and better reading ability.

There are numerous reports, extending over more than 100 years, of an association of greater myopia prevalence with higher educational attainment and occupations having heavier near work demands (Curtin, 1985; Adams et al., 1989; Ong and Ciuffreda, 1997). For example, in an extensive epidemiologic survey, Goldschmidt (1968) found higher prevalences of myopia in Denmark in persons with occupations requiring more near work. Richler and Bear (1980) found that correlations of refractive error and time spent on near work remained significant after controlling for age, sex, and level of education.

Krause et al. (1982) found higher myopia prevalence in those patients with higher socioeconomic status in Finland. Rosner and Belkin (1987) found that greater intelligence and more years of school were related to myopia prevalence in 17- to 19-year-old males in Israel. Two studies found higher myopia prevalence in urban dwellers than in persons from rural areas (Jain et al., 1983; Paritsis et al., 1983), but one study did not demonstrate that result (Angle and Wissman, 1980).

Some startlingly high myopia prevalences have been reported in Asia. Ko (1984) reported prevalences of 81–89% in high school students in the cities of Taipei and Koahshiung in Taiwan; Lin et al. (1988) gave a prevalence of 75% among schoolchildren 18 years of age in Taiwan. Rajan et al. (1998) reported myopia prevalence to be 51.5% in a sample of 12-year-olds in Singapore. A Japanese study gave myopia prevalences of 51% in 1985 and 68% in 1995 for students in their third year of high school (Hirai et al., 1998), and among 12-year-olds in Hong Kong, prevalences of 55–58% were reported (Edwards, 1998).

Classification of Myopia

Grosvenor (1987) reviewed several different systems of classifying myopia. Different authors have classified myopia according to whether it is stationary or progressive, amount of myopia, presumed cause, optical correlate (e.g., axial or refractive), and various combinations thereof. Problems with all these classification systems include ambiguity in where cutoff values should be (as in classification by amount) and difficulty in obtaining and verifying the information necessary to make a categorization. Grosvenor proposed that a much simplified and more easily verifiable system would be to classify myopia on the basis of age-related prevalence and age of onset. The prevalence data compiled in Tables 1.6–1.9 were used to arrive at the following four categories:

1. *Congenital myopia* is present at birth and persists through the emmetropization period of infancy; it is present when a child enters school. The amount of myopia is high enough that it is usually present throughout life. The prevalence of this form of myopia is 1–2%.

2. *Youth-onset myopia* has its onset between about age 5 or 6 years and physical maturity in the mid- to late teens. This is the most common

type of myopia. Myopia prevalence in the United States increases from 1% to 2% at approximately age 6 years to approximately 25% in the late teens.

3. *Early adult–onset myopia* has its onset after physical maturity is reached and before approximately age 40 years. Myopia prevalence increases over these years, reaching 30–35% at age 40 years in the United States.

4. *Late adult–onset myopia* has its onset after age 40 years. Figure 1.1 is a graphic representation of myopia prevalence as a function of age and Grosvenor's (1987) classification system.

Another classification scheme is to categorize myopia by clinical entity (Goss and Eskridge, 1987). These categories are simple myopia, night myopia, pseudomyopia, pathologic myopia, and induced myopia. *Simple myopia* is characterized by normal visual acuity with optical correction and an absence of obvious structural anomalies of the eye other than small simple myopic temporal crescents. It is by far the most common type of myopia. *Night myopia* is a shift toward myopia in low illumination or darkness due to the dark focus of accommodation. *Pseudomyopia* is an apparent myopia due to unrelaxed accommodation and is diagnosed by finding minus or more minus on manifest refraction, compared with plus or a lesser amount of minus on cycloplegic refraction. *Pathologic myopia* is a high myopia associated with pathologic or degenerative changes in the posterior segment of the eye. *Induced myopia* is myopia induced by external factors affecting the eye, such as inadvertent exposure to pharmaceutic agents that increase accommodation, or by internal changes, such as blood sugar fluctuations in diabetes. This book deals mainly with simple myopia and, to a lesser extent, pathologic myopia. Night myopia, pseudomyopia, and induced myopia are discussed in Chapter 4.

Curtin (1985) has recognized that simple myopia and pathologic myopia may be considered as a continuum, and has proposed that an inter-

FIGURE 1.1. Graphic representation of the prevalence of myopia (–0.50 D or greater) with age, classified as congenital, youth-onset, early adult–onset, and late adult–onset. (Reprinted with permission from T Grosvenor. A review and a suggested classification system for myopia on the basis of age-related prevalence and age of onset. Am J Optom Physiol Opt 1987;64:545–554.)

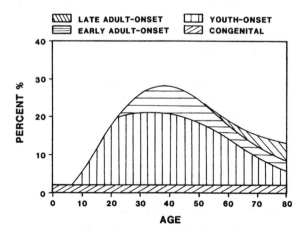

TABLE 1.11
Prevalence of Myopia as a Function of Parental History of Myopia from Different Studies: Percentage of Children with Myopia

Study	Parents Myopic					
	Neither Parent	Only Father	Only Mother	One Parent	One or Both Parents	Both Parents
Paul (1938)	10%			30%		60%
Wold (1949)	35%				49%	
Keller (1973)	15%			40%		45%
Ashton (JA) (1985)	11%	17%	25%			46%
Ashton (EA) (1985)	11%	16%	24%			33%
Gwiazda et al. (1993)	8%			23%		42%
Zadnik et al. (1994)	2%			5%		11%
Quinn et al.* (1995)	21%				30%	
Goss and Jackson (1996c)	6%	42%	35%	37%	43%	57%

JA = Japanese ancestry; EA = European ancestry.
*Right eyes.

mediate myopia could be described. Curtin defined *simple* or *physiologic myopia* to be a low myopia (approximately –3 D or less) with no fundus changes. In *intermediate myopia*, there is a moderate amount of myopia (–3 to –5 D) and temporal crescents are present. Curtin considers *pathologic myopia* to be a high myopia in which ocular complications, especially posterior segment anomalies, result from excessive axial elongation.

Risk Factors for Myopia Onset

One way to imply risk is to look at factors that are related to higher prevalence. One such factor is near work. The possible role of near work in the development of myopia is discussed in Chapter 2.

A positive family history of myopia is a risk factor for myopia. Several studies, summarized in Table 1.11, have found that myopia is most likely to occur when both parents are myopic and least likely when neither parent is myopic. Although this may be due, in large part, to inheritance, the influence of common environment and lifestyle factors in parents and offspring cannot be ruled out.

A refractive error of emmetropia or very low hyperopia, as opposed to higher amounts of hyperopia, is a risk factor for myopia. Hirsch (1964) did

TABLE 1.12
Refractive Error at Age 13 or 14 Years as a Function of Refractive at Age 5 or 6

Spherical Equivalent Refraction at Age 5–6	Spherical Equivalent Refraction at Age 13–14		
	Myopia (≥–0.50 D)	Emmetropia* (–0.49 to +0.99 D)	Hyperopia (≥1.00 D)
>–0.26 D	4	0	0
–0.25 to –0.01 D	6	0	0
0.00 to +0.24 D	7	6	0
+0.25 to + 0.49 D	37	4	0
+0.50 to +0.74 D	21	33	5
+0.75 to +0.99 D	15	41	10
+1.00 to +1.24 D	2	15	14
+1.25 to +1.49 D	0	1	7
>+1.50 D	0	0	33
Total	92	100	69

*The 100 with emmetropia at age 13 or 14 in the table were randomly selected from a total of 605 with emmetropia at that age.
Source: Data from MJ Hirsch. Predictability of refraction at age 14 on the basis of testing at age 6—interim report from the Ojai longitudinal study of refraction. Am J Optom Arch Am Acad Optom 1964;41:567–573.

manifest retinoscopy as part of a twice-yearly school screening in southern California. Because he continued these measurements for several years, he had extensive longitudinal data. He tabulated refractive error at age 13 or 14 years as a function of refractive error at age 5 or 6, for 766 eyes of 383 children, randomly selecting 100 of the 605 emmetropic eyes for his analysis. The data he presented are summarized in Table 1.12. Based on these data and assuming that the numbers in the emmetropia column should be multiplied by about six, we can suggest some conclusions about predictability of refractive errors at age 13 or 14 years from refraction at age 5 or 6 years:

1. Children with hyperopia of +1.50 D or more at age 5 or 6 years are likely to still be hyperopic at age 13 or 14 years.
2. Many children in the +0.50 to +1.24 D range at age 5 or 6 years will be in the emmetropic range (defined as –0.49 to +0.99 D by Hirsch).
3. Many children who have refractions between 0 and +0.49 D at age 5 or 6 years will be myopic at age 13 or 14 years.
4. Children who are myopic at age 5 or 6 years will become more myopic by age 13 or 14 years.

Hirsch also found that children with against-the-rule astigmatism were more likely to become myopic than children with no astigmatism or with-the-rule astigmatism.

Gwiazda et al. (1993), in a study conducted in Boston, presented manifest refraction data for 72 children tested before age 6 months and fol-

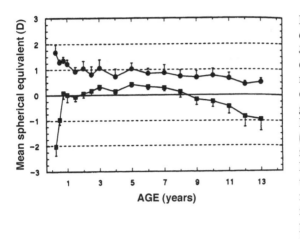

FIGURE 1.2. Mean spherical equivalent refractive error for 31 children with minus spherical equivalents before 6 months of age and for 20 children with spherical equivalents greater than or equal to +0.50 D before 6 months of age. (Reprinted with permission from J Gwiazda, F Thorn, J Bauer, R Held. Emmetropization and the progression of manifest refraction in children followed from infancy to puberty. Clin Vis Sci 1993; 8:337–344.)

lowed for at least 9 years. They observed that both hyperopic and myopic infants shift toward emmetropia in the first few months of life. An interesting finding, not previously reported, was that 42% of the children who were myopic as infants and became emmetropic or hyperopic by age 3 years again became myopic by age 8 or 9 years. In comparison, only 10% of the children who were hyperopic as infants became myopic during the same period. This difference is reflected in the changes in mean refractive errors for initially myopic and initially hyperopic infants in Figure 1.2.

Mutti and Zadnik (1995) used Bayesian analysis to compare prediction of myopia from refractive error at school entry, refraction in infancy, and parental history of myopia. Data on school entry were taken from Hirsch (1964), data on refractive error in infancy were taken from Gwiazda et al. (1993), and the parental history data were taken from their own longitudinal study (Zadnik et al., 1993). *Refractive error at school entry* was a much better predictor of myopia than was either refractive error in infancy or parental history. Several studies have reported higher intraocular pressures (IOPs) in myopic eyes than in nonmyopic eyes (Abdalla and Hamdi, 1970; Tomlinson and Phillips, 1970; Edwards and Brown, 1993; Quinn et al., 1995). This association is consistent with theories suggesting that increased IOP is a cause of myopia (Young, 1975, 1977; Pruett, 1988; Greene, 1991; Young and Leary, 1991). However, Edwards and Brown (1996) found that IOP was not high before myopia onset in Chinese children 7 years of age or older, but rather increased *after* myopia onset. Thirteen children who became myopic had mean IOPs of 13.4 mm Hg before myopia onset, and 14.6 mm Hg after myopia onset. Goss and Caffey (submitted manuscript) also found IOP was not higher in children who became myopic than in children who did not. Myopia may be a risk factor for an increase in IOP, rather than increased IOP being a risk factor for myopia.

TABLE 1.13
Summary of Clinical Test Results in Persons Who Became Myopic
Compared with Persons Who Did Not

	Dynamic Retinoscopy	Near Binocular Cross Cylinder	Positive Relative Accommodation	Near Phoria
Became myopic group				
n	24	18	20	23
Mean	+1.28 D	+1.33 D	–2.84 D	+0.59Δ
SD	0.72	0.57	1.89	6.73
Remained emmetropic group				
n	25	18	24	23
Mean	+0.79 D	+0.82 D	–4.02 D	–2.3Δ
SD	0.81	0.52	1.95	4.16
Statistical significance of difference by t-test (p)	0.03	0.008	0.04	0.08

SD = standard deviation.
Source: Data from B Drobe, R de Saint-André. The pre-myopic syndrome. Ophthal Physiol Opt 1995;5:375–378.

Goss (1991a) collected records from seven optometry practices of 75 children who became myopic and their emmetropic matches by age, gender, and clinic location. The mean nearpoint von Graefe phorias were 1.0Δ esophoria (SD = 6.0) for children who became myopic and 2.0Δ exophoria (SD = 6.0) for children who remained emmetropic. The difference was statistically significant (p <.001). The mean near binocular cross-cylinder findings were +0.90 D (SD = 0.49) in the group that became myopic and +0.72 D (SD = 0.50) in the remained emmetropic group. The difference in binocular cross-cylinder findings between groups was statistically significant by analysis of variance when the effect of location was taken into account. Positive relative accommodation averaged –2.53 D (n = 32, SD = 0.98) in the group that became myopic and –3.16 D (n = 32, SD = 1.03) in the remaining emmetropic group. This difference was statistically significant (p <.02). However, negative relative accommodation was not significantly different in the two groups.

Very similar results, summarized in Table 1.13, were obtained by Drobe and de Saint-André (1995). They compared test findings in 25 patients younger than age 40 years who became myopic (mean age, 12.77 years) to a like number of patients also younger than age 40 years who remained emmetropic (mean age, 13.76 years). The patients who eventually became myopic were initially found to accept more plus on both dynamic

TABLE 1.14
Means and Standard Deviations for Keratometer Power in Children Who Became
Myopic and Children Who Did Not

	Right Eye Horizontal Keratometry		Right Eye Vertical Keratometry	
	Males	*Females*	*Males*	*Females*
Became myopic group				
n	15	14	15	14
Mean (D)	43.83	44.63	44.36	45.22
SD	1.14	1.76	1.31	1.52
Remained emmetropic group				
n	27	31	27	31
Mean (D)	43.12	43.85	43.42	44.39
SD	1.77	1.56	1.83	1.78

SD = standard deviation.
Source: Data from DA Goss, TW Jackson. Clinical findings before the onset of myopia in youth. 1. Ocular optical components. Optom Vis Sci 1995;72:870–878.

retinoscopy and the near binocular cross-cylinder test and to have lower positive relative accommodation. The mean horizontal phorias were 0.59 esophoria in the group that became myopic and 2.3 exophoria in the remaining emmetropic group. The difference in phorias was not quite statistically significant at the 0.05 level, but the magnitudes of the values and of the difference were very similar to those found by Goss (1991a).

Goss and Jackson (1995; 1996a,b,c) conducted a prospective longitudinal study in which they followed a cohort of initially emmetropic children for 3 years. Test findings were compared in 29 children who became myopic (age range, 9.1–14.3 years) with 58 children who remained emmetropic (age range, 8.5–13.8 years). The axial length–to–corneal radius ratio (AL/CR) was significantly higher in the group that became myopic than in the remaining emmetropic group ($p < .001$). The horizontal meridian AL/CR was 3.00 or greater in 88% of the group that became myopic (sensitivity = 0.88), and was less than 3.00 in 68% of the remaining emmetropic group (specificity = 0.68). Axial length was not significantly different in the two groups. Corneal power was greater in the children who became myopic than in the children who remained emmetropic ($p < .05$ for the horizontal meridian and $p < .03$ for the vertical meridian). Therefore, both the AL/CR ratio and corneal power (alone) were risk factors for myopia. Keratometer findings for the two groups are summarized in Table 1.14.

Goss and Jackson (1996a,b) also presented data on accommodation and vergence. As the studies by Goss (1991a) and by Drobe and de Saint-André (1995) indicate, the positive relative accommodation was lower in the became myopic group ($p < .02$). In an analysis of fusional vergence data, Goss and Jackson (1996a) found the midpoint of the near fusional vergence range to be more convergent in the group that became myopic (mean, +5.8) than in the remaining emmetropic group (mean, +3.2). The difference is significant at the 0.004 level. The mean near phorias were not significantly different in the two groups (Goss and Jackson, 1996b). There were, however, proportionately more subjects who became myopic outside the range of 3 exophoria to 1 esophoria than remaining emmetropic subjects (p <.05 on chi-square test). In the Goss (1991a) and Drobe and de Saint-André (1995) studies, *esophoria* was a risk factor for myopia. In the Goss and Jackson (1996b) data, it appeared that *both esophoria and higher exophorias* were risk factors for myopia.

An interesting finding from Goss and Jackson (1996b) was a convergent shift in the near phoria in the children who became myopic. A mean shift of more than 3Δ occurred over approximately 2.5 years, beginning before myopia onset and continuing afterward. A very similar shift was found when they examined the private practice data set previously collected by Goss (1991a). Furthermore, a shift in near phoria was not found in the remained emmetropic groups from either study.

Summary of Risk Factors for Myopia

Cross-sectional studies have shown that factors associated with higher prevalences of myopia include occupations requiring higher levels of near work, higher educational status, and higher socioeconomic status. Prevalence may also be somewhat higher among females and urban dwellers.

Longitudinal studies have identified some additional risk factors. These include (1) positive family history of myopia, (2) myopia in infancy, (3) refractive error of emmetropia or hyperopia less than +0.50 D at school entry, (4) esophoria, (5) low positive-relative accommodation, (6) more plus on near binocular cross-cylinder test, (7) high AL/CR, and (8) higher corneal power.

Progression of Myopia

It is known that once myopia appears in childhood, it inevitably increases in amount (Goss, 1991b). Progression of myopia in young adulthood is also common, but generally not as great in magnitude as in childhood (Adams et al., 1989).

Patterns of Childhood Myopia Progression

Typical myopia progression patterns are illustrated in Figures 1.3 and 1.4. Additional typical cases in which refractions were performed both before and after the onset of myopia are shown in Figure 1.5. These plots clearly show that refractive change accelerates as a child crosses the line from zero refractive error into myopia.

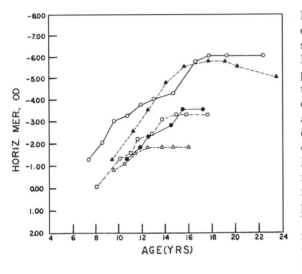

FIGURE 1.3. Typical patterns of childhood myopia progression. Data are from five males. Refractive error in the principal meridian nearest horizontal in the right eye is plotted on the y-axis as a function of age on the x-axis. Each set of common symbols represents data for one person. (HORIZ. MER., OD = principal meridian nearest horizontal in the right eye.) (Reprinted with permission from DA Goss, RL Winkler. Progression of myopia in youth: age of cessation. Am J Optom Physiol Opt 1983;60:651–658.)

Rates of childhood myopia progression show considerable individual variation. Goss and Cox (1985) calculated rates using linear regression analysis for myopic children who had four or more manifest subjective refractions between the ages of 6 and 15 years. Data were collected from five optometry practices in the central United States. The mean rate of myopia progression for girls was –0.43 D per year (n = 145, SD = 0.25), and the mean rate for boys was –0.40 D per year (n = 158, SD = 0.24). The distribution of rates of progression is shown in Table 1.15.

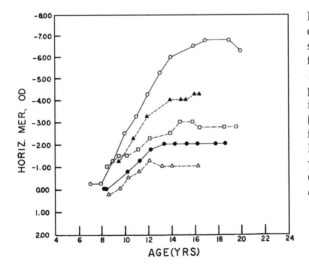

FIGURE 1.4. Typical patterns of childhood myopia progression. Data are from five females. Axes are as in Figure 1.3. (HORIZ. MER., OD = principal meridian nearest horizontal in the right eye.) (Reprinted with permission from DA Goss, RL Winkler. Progression of myopia in youth: age of cessation. Am J Optom Physiol Opt 1983;60: 651–658.)

FIGURE 1.5. Typical patterns of childhood myopia progression illustrating the acceleration of refractive change at the onset of myopia. Axes are as in Figure 1.3. (HORIZ. MER. OD = principal meridian nearest horizontal in the right eye.) (Reprinted with permission from DA Goss. Linearity of refractive change with age in childhood myopia progression. Am J Optom Physiol Opt 1987;64:775–780.)

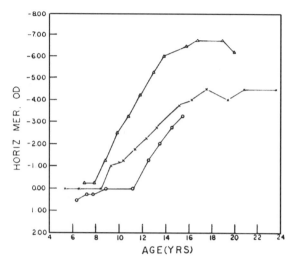

Progression rates were calculated by Mäntyjärvi (1985a) from cycloplegic retinoscopy data for myopic children examined at a community health center in Finland. Children were examined initially at age 5–8 years and were followed up to age 15 years. The mean progression rate was –0.55 D per year (n = 133, SD = 0.27). The range of rates was from 0 to –1.63 D per year. Mean rates of progression for various studies in the United States and Europe have been between –0.3 and –0.6 D per year (Baldwin et al., 1969; Goss, 1984, 1990, 1994; Mäntyjärvi, 1985a; Grosvenor et al., 1987;

TABLE 1.15
Frequency Distribution of Childhood Myopia Progression Rates

Rates (D/year)	Number of Males	Number of Females
+0.20 to 0.00	0	4 (2.8%)
–0.01 to –0.20	37 (23.4%)	20 (13.8%)
–0.21 to –0.40	51 (32.3%)	48 (33.1%)
–0.41 to –0.60	41 (25.9%)	44 (30.3%)
–0.61 to –0.80	15 (9.5%)	23 (15.9%)
–0.81 to –1.00	12 (7.6%)	7 (4.8%)
–1.01 to –1.20	2 (1.3%)	1 (0.7%)
–1.21 to –1.40	0	0
–1.41 to –1.60	0	1 (0.7%)
Total	158 (100%)	145 (100%)

Source: Reprinted with permission from DA Goss, VD Cox. Trends in the change of clinical refractive error in myopes. J Am Optom Assoc 1985;56:608–613.

Jensen, 1991). Mean childhood myopia progression rates reported from different studies in Japan have ranged from –0.5 to –0.8 D per year (Tokoro and Kabe, 1964a,b, 1965; Matsuo, 1965; Otsuka, 1967). Tsai et al. (1998) reported a mean progression rate of –0.64 D per year in Taiwan.

Childhood myopia progression typically slows or stops in the mid- to late teenage years. Goss and Winkler (1983) used four related mathematical methods to derive an index of the *age of cessation* of childhood myopia progression. Manifest subjective refraction data were collected from three optometry practices in the midwestern United States. One method for derivation of cessation age involved determining the best fitting straight line through points between 6 and 15 years. The age at which that line reached the amount of myopia that the patient averaged at examinations after the age of 17 years was the cessation age. The mean cessation age for females was 15.21 years ($n = 57$, SD = 1.74), and the mean cessation age for males was 16.66 years ($n = 66$, SD = 2.10). These are approximately the ages of the end of the adolescent growth spurt (Lowrey, 1978). Cessation ages for males and females were significantly different ($p < .0001$). The standard deviations of approximately 2 years indicate quite a bit of individual variability in cessation age.

Factors Affecting Rates of Childhood Myopia Progression

Higher progression rates are associated with earlier onset of myopia (Bücklers, 1953; Rosenberg and Goldschmidt, 1981; Fledelius, 1981; Grosvenor et al., 1987; Goss, 1990). However, no correlation between myopia onset age and cessation age has been observed (Goss and Cox, 1985). As a result of the higher rate and because progression continues over a longer period, earlier onset of myopia results in a higher amount of myopia in the late teens or early adulthood (Francois and Goes, 1975; Lecaillon-Thibon, 1981; Septon, 1984; Mäntyjärvi, 1985b; Goss and Cox, 1985). For example, data from Mäntyjärvi (1985b) are shown in Table 1.16.

Higher progression rates not surprisingly have been found to be related to greater time spent on near work. Pärssinen et al. (1989) conducted a study in Finland in which myopic children were examined at age 9–11 years and then followed for 3 years. The subjects and their parents completed questionnaires that included questions about reading and near work. Refractive error change and amount of time spent reading and doing near work showed a weak but statistically significant correlation ($r = -0.25$, $p < .001$). Higher amounts of myopia progression showed a weak correlation with shorter reading distance ($r = +0.22$, $p < .001$). Higher progression was also correlated with less time spent outdoors ($r = +0.17$, $p = .004$). Jensen (1991) did not find a difference in myopia progression in 2 years between Danish schoolchildren who averaged 2 or more hours reading per day and those who did not. Two studies found greater myopia pro-

TABLE 1.16
Mean Amount of Myopia at Age 15 or 16 Years as a Function
of Age of Myopia Onset

| Age of Myopia Onset (years) | Refractive Error at 15–16 Years | | |
	Number of Children	Mean	SD
7–10	40	–4.46	1.63
11–13	122	–2.87	1.15
14–15	52	–1.66	1.00

Source: Reprinted with permission from MI Mäntyjärvi. Predicting of myopia progression in school children. J Pediatr Ophthalmol Strab 1985;22:71–75.

gression rates in a 6-month period during the school year than in a 6-month period that included the summer vacation (Fulk and Cyert, 1996; Goss and Rainey, 1998).

Two studies did not find a relation of type or amount of astigmatism with myopia progression rates (Goss and Shewey, 1990; Pärssinen, 1991). Jensen (1991, 1992) found greater myopia progression in 2 years in Danish children with higher IOP and in children with temporal pigment crescents at the optic nerve head. Twenty-seven children who had IOPs higher than 16 mm Hg at age 9–12 years had an average myopia progression of –1.32 D over the next 2 years. Twenty children with IOPs of 16 mm Hg or less had an average myopia progression of –0.86 D, and 28 children who started the study with pigment crescents had an average myopia of –3.26 D at the beginning of the study with mean progression of –1.39 D in 2 years. Twenty-one children without crescents started at –2.20 D of myopia and progressed an additional –0.81 D in 2 years.

Higher childhood myopia rates have been reported to be associated with esophoria at near. Roberts and Banford (1963, 1967) calculated myopia progression rates from manifest subjective refraction data for children seen in their optometry practices in New York. Near phorias were determined using the von Graefe prism dissociation technique with a fixation target at 40 cm. The mean progression rate for 76 children with exophoria greater than 4Δ was –0.43 D per year. The mean rate for 105 children with near phorias between ortho and 4Δ exophoria was –0.39 D per year. The average rate for 167 patients with esophoria was –0.48 D per year. Progression rates increased as the amount of esophoria increased. Goss (1990) used manifest subjective refractions from four optometry practices and two longitudinal university studies to calculate myopia progression rates by linear regression. For children who had a habitual near phoria greater than 6Δ exophoria, the mean myopia progres-

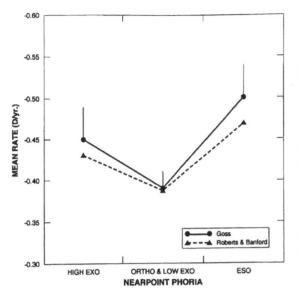

FIGURE 1.6. Mean rates of childhood myopia progression as a function of near phoria determined by the von Graefe method, data from Roberts and Banford (1963, 1967) and Goss (1990). The ortho and low exophoria category ranged from 0 to 4Δ exophoria in the Roberts and Banford study and from 0 to 6Δ exophoria in the Goss study. Error bars represent one standard error. (Reprinted with permission from DA Goss. Effect of spectacle correction on the progression of myopia in children—a literature review. J Am Optom Assoc 1994;65:117–128.)

sion rate was –0.45 D per year (*n* = 67, SD = 0.27). The mean progression rate for habitual near phorias in the range of ortho to 6Δ exophoria was –0.39 D per year (*n* = 110, SD = 0.25). The average rate for children with esophoria at near through their habitual correction was –0.50 D per year (*n* = 77, SD = 0.32). The rates in the three groups were significantly different by analysis of variance (*p* <.025). The results of these two studies are very similar and are illustrated in Figure 1.6. The progression rates were lowest when near phorias were normal (normal range for near phorias being ortho to 6Δ exophoria in the norms published by Morgan, 1944), rates were a little higher in cases with higher exophoria, and rates were highest in esophoria.

To summarize the studies on factors affecting childhood myopia progression rates, higher rates are associated with earlier onset age, greater amount of time spent on reading and near work, shorter reading distance, less time spent outdoors, higher IOP, presence of temporal pigment crescents, and esophoria at near.

Ocular Optical Component Changes in Childhood Myopia Progression

The ocular optical component change that produces the increases in myopia in childhood is axial elongation of the vitreous chamber. Data from Sorsby and Leary (1970) illustrating the correlation of increase in axial length of the eye with myopia progression are given in Figure 1.7.

FIGURE 1.7. Amount of myopia progression as a function of axial elongation of the eye in 25 children in England from the data of Sorsby and Leary (1970). (Reprinted with permission from T Grosvenor. Primary Care Optometry: Anomalies of Refraction and Binocular Vision [3rd ed]. Boston: Butterworth–Heinemann, 1996;46.)

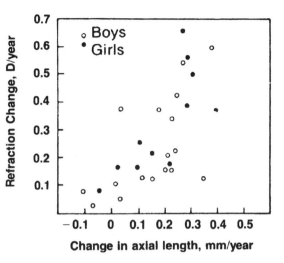

Data from Tokoro and Kabe (1964b) in Table 1.17 show an increase in axial length, a decrease in crystalline lens power, and a negligible change in corneal power in childhood myopia progression.

Fledelius (1981) reported on refractive changes between ages 10 and 18 years in 137 Danes, 45% of whom were myopic. Seventy of the subjects had been born with low birth weight; 67 had been born full-term. The correlations of change in refractive error and change in vitreous depth were found to be high: $r = -0.76$ in the full-term group and $r = -0.62$ in the low-birth-weight group. All these findings indicate the ocular optical compo-

TABLE 1.17
Mean Changes in Refractive Error and Ocular Optical Components in 1 Year in Myopes in Japan

Age Span (years)	Number of Eyes	Change in Refractive Error (D)	Change in Corneal Power (D)	Change in Crystalline Lens Power (D)	Change in Axial Length (mm)
7–10	18	–0.60 (0.27)	–0.06 (0.08)	–0.36 (0.31)	+0.32 (0.11)
11–15	15	–0.70 (0.38)	–0.03 (0.08)	–0.23 (0.15)	+0.32 (0.16)
16–22	9	–0.13 (0.15)	–0.02 (0.16)	–0.05 (0.19)	+0.03 (0.04)

Standard deviations are given in parentheses.
Source: Data from T Tokoro, S Kabe. Treatment of myopia and the changes in optical components. Report I. Topical application of Neosynephrine and tropicamide. Acta Soc Ophthalmol Jpn 1964;68:1958–1961.

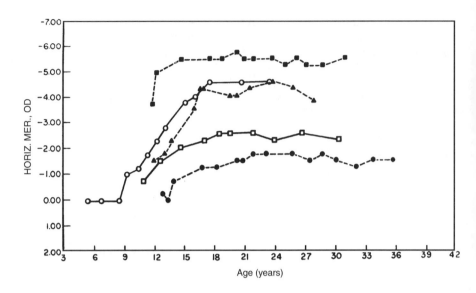

FIGURE 1.8. Examples of adult stabilization of myopia progression, in which there is little or no increase in myopia in young adulthood after childhood myopia progression. Refractive error in the principal meridian nearest horizontal in the right eye is plotted as a function of age. (HORIZ. MER., OD = principal meridian nearest horizontal in the right eye.) (Reprinted with permission from DA Goss, P Erickson, VD Cox. Prevalence and pattern of adult myopia progression in a general optometric practice. Am J Optom Physiol Opt 1985;62:470–477.)

nent change responsible for childhood myopia progression is axial elongation through increase in vitreous depth.

Patterns of Young Adulthood Myopia Progression

The most common form of myopia in Grosvenor's (1987) myopia classification system is youth-onset myopia, and the second most common is early adult–onset myopia (see Figure 1.1). The young adult years can also be a time when youth-onset myopes have further, but usually slower, increases in their myopia. In a survey of optometrists, Grosvenor (1977) found the average myopia progression between ages 20 and 40 years for persons who were myopic at age 20 was approximately –1.00 D, or approximately –0.05 D per year.

Goss et al. (1985) collected longitudinal records from five optometry practices in the central United States. By comparing childhood myopia progression and young adulthood myopia progression in 116 cases in which longitudinal refractive data extended over many years, they defined three basic patterns, which they called *adult stabilization, adult continuation,* and *adult acceleration.* Examples of these patterns are shown in Figures 1.8–1.10. *Adult stabilization,* characterized by stabilization of

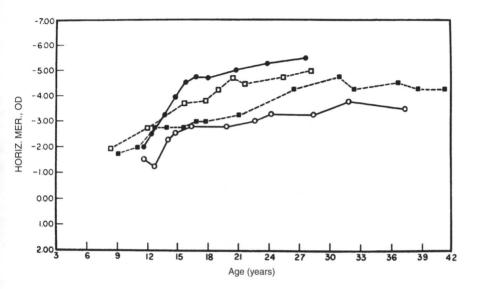

FIGURE 1.9. Examples of adult continuation of myopia progression, in which myopia progression continues in young adulthood after progression in childhood, but at a lower rate. Refractive error in the principal meridian nearest horizontal in the right eye is plotted as a function of age. (HORIZ. MER., OD = principal meridian nearest horizontal in the right eye.) (Reprinted with permission from DA Goss, P Erickson, VD Cox. Prevalence and pattern of adult myopia progression in a general optometric practice. Am J Optom Physiol Opt 1985;62:470–477.)

myopia in young adulthood after childhood progression, was found in 87% of females and 68% of males. *Adult continuation,* in which myopia progression continues in young adulthood at a slower rate than in childhood, was found in 13% of females and 25% of males. In *adult acceleration,* myopia has its onset in young adulthood (Grosvenor's early adult–onset myopia classification), or youth-onset myopia progresses faster in young adulthood than in childhood. Adult acceleration was not found in any of the 53 females in the sample, but was found in 6% of the 63 males. Most of the persons in the adult continuation and adult acceleration categories had myopia progression rates between –0.05 and –0.20 D per year. Higher young adulthood myopia progression has been reported for persons in graduate school and in military academies (Dunphy et al., 1968; Sutton and Ditmars, 1970; O'Neal and Connon, 1987; Zadnik and Mutti, 1987; Adams et al., 1989).

Ocular Optical Component Changes in Young Adulthood Myopia Progression

Three studies have compared one-time component measurements in small groups of young adult emmetropes and early adult–onset myopes (Grosvenor,

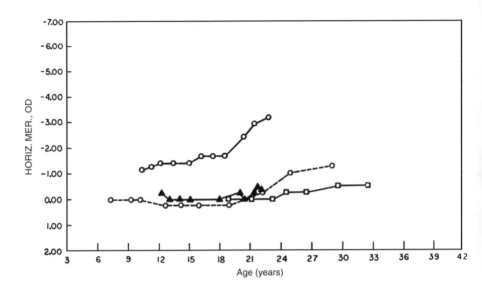

FIGURE 1.10. Examples of adult acceleration of myopia progression, in which myopia has its onset in young adulthood or progresses at a faster rate in young adulthood than in childhood. Refractive error in the principal meridian nearest horizontal in the right eye is plotted as a function of age. (HORIZ. MER., OD = principal meridian nearest horizontal in the right eye.) (Reprinted with permission from DA Goss, P Erickson, VD Cox. Prevalence and pattern of adult myopia progression in a general optometric practice. Am J Optom Physiol Opt 1985;62:470–477.)

1994). McBrien and Millodot (1987) reported greater anterior chamber depth, lesser crystalline lens thickness, and greater vitreous depth in the myopes than in the emmetropes. Grosvenor and Scott (1991) found the cornea to be more powerful in early adult–onset myopes than in emmetropes. Bullimore et al. (1992) found early adult–onset myopes to have greater vitreous depths than emmetropes.

Longitudinal keratometer data from optometry patient files have shown corneal steepening in young adulthood myopia progression (Baldwin, 1962; Kent, 1963; Goss and Erickson, 1987). For example, Goss and Erickson (1987) calculated rates of young adulthood myopia progression and rates of corneal power change by linear regression. For the principal meridian nearest vertical, the correlation coefficients between myopia progression rates and corneal power change rates were $+0.66$ ($n = 22$, $p < .001$) in males and $+0.69$ ($n = 15$, $p < .005$) in females. For the horizontal meridian, the coefficients of correlation were $+0.29$ (not significant at the 0.05 level) for males and $+0.58$ ($p < .05$) for females. Although the correlations were significant, the amounts of corneal steepening were fairly low, so that the cornea could not have been the main contributor to myopia progression.

Two longitudinal prospective studies have provided vitreous depth data. Grosvenor and Scott (1993) found that the progression of myopia over a 3-year period in 16 early adult–onset myopes was correlated with increases in vitreous depth (r = –0.77). Grosvenor and Scott did not find a significant correlation of myopia progression and corneal power change. McBrien and Adams (1997) followed a group of 251 clinical microscopists (ages, 21–63 years) for 2 years. The only statistically significant ocular optical component change noted for those with myopia progression was an increase in vitreous depth.

Based on the available studies, it appears that young adulthood myopia progression is produced mainly by vitreous depth increases with a slight contribution from corneal steepening. It is possible that some longitudinal studies have failed to find the small corneal contribution because it may have been masked by averaging principal meridians rather than by performing separate meridional analyses (Grosvenor and Goss, 1998).

Pathologic Changes in Myopia

Many of the pathologic changes that may be found in a myopic eye occur *only* in myopic eyes, whereas other pathologic changes can occur in any eye regardless of refractive error but have a greater prevalence—or more serious consequences—in myopic eyes. Pathologic changes in myopic eyes may be conveniently discussed in terms of those affecting the central (posterior) fundus and those affecting the peripheral (anterior) fundus.

Central Fundus

The pathologic changes most commonly seen in the central (posterior) fundus include optic nerve crescents, myopic cupping of the disk, posterior staphyloma formation, and chorioretinal changes, including retinal hemorrhages, lacquer cracks, and chorioretinal atrophy. More severe pathologic changes that may be found in the higher degrees of myopia, particularly during the adult years, include progression of existing optic nerve changes and staphylomas, subretinal neovascularization, and Fuchs' spot.

Optic Nerve Crescents

One of the earliest fundus changes in the myopic eye is the presence of an optic nerve crescent, also called a *scleral crescent*, a *temporal crescent*, or *myopic conus*, which is due to a pulling away of the choroid and pigment epithelium from the optic nerve head, usually on the temporal side, allowing scleral tissue to be seen. Closely related to a scleral crescent is a *choroidal crescent*, which is characterized by the presence of choroidal vessels and pigment in the crescent area. According to Perkins (1981), a scleral or choroidal crescent is generally present in myopia of –4.00 D or more.

Repeated examinations of a large number of myopic children, ages 8–15 years, in two myopia control studies (Grosvenor et al., 1987, 1991), resulted in the clinical impression that in this age group eyes with myopia of –3.00 D or greater almost always developed an optic nerve crescent, whereas eyes with myopia no greater than –1.00 or –1.50 D seldom had crescents.

Fulk et al. (1992) used stereophotography to study optic nerve crescents in the eyes of 224 subjects ages 8–25 years, 55% of whom were myopes. For each photograph, the horizontal dimension of the crescent, if any, was measured in tenths of millimeters. Although some crescents were as wide as 0.675 mm, the majority were no wider than 0.3 mm, with the greatest frequency being 0.125 mm. Crescent width was found to be associated with the amount of myopia ($p <.0001$): the greater the amount of myopia, the wider the crescent. Fulk et al. concluded, "The presence of a crescent in a young myope may be clinically important in that it may indicate a risk for more rapid increase in myopia as the child grows."

It is worthy of emphasis that although some authors have suggested that the presence of a crescent depends more on increased axial length than on the magnitude of myopia, Fulk et al. (1992) found that once refractive error was accounted for, axial length provided no additional information concerning the presence or absence of a crescent. They suggested that if an eye attains a longer than normal axial length due to normal growth, it is not likely to develop a crescent, but if the increased length results in myopia, it is more likely to have a crescent. This is consistent with the finding (Grosvenor and Scott, 1994) that axial length is less highly correlated with refractive error than the AL/CR ratio. For a group of 149 young adults between 18 and 34 years of age, the correlation between refractive error and axial length was found to be 0.76, but the correlation between refractive error and the AL/CR ratio was found to be 0.92. These correlations indicate that whereas axial length accounts for 58% of the variance in refractive error, the AL/CR ratio accounts for 85% of the variance.

Myopic Disk Cupping

Almost 100 years ago—long before the term *cup/disk ratio* was coined— Elschnig described five types of cupping that can occur in the optic nerve head. As described in some detail by Kronfeld (1951) and Shlaifer (1959), a type I optic nerve head is essentially flat, with no cupping; types II and III are cylindrical and saucer-shaped physiologic cups; type IV is a myopic cup; and type V includes a number of categories including the glaucomatous cup. Type IV is described as the typical myopic cupping: The retinal arteries and veins are pushed toward the nasal border of the disk, and a rather wide and deep cup is present, having its greatest depth nasally and becoming increasingly shallow temporally. There may be a displacement of the retinal and choroidal tissue over the nasal surface of the optic nerve, known as *nasal supertraction*. A common observation, confirmed by Carpel and Engstrom (1981) is that the cup/disk ratio is significantly larger than normal only in *moderate* myopia. A possible explanation for this is that in higher degrees of myopia the formation of a posterior staphyloma alters the mechanical forces at the posterior pole in such a way that optic disk cupping is no longer present.

A problem presented by myopic disk cupping is that its appearance is very much like that of *glaucomatous* cupping: If a practitioner's mindset is to be concerned only with a high cup/disk ratio in a myopic eye, it is possible that cases of open-angle glaucoma could be missed.

Posterior Staphyloma Formation

As described by Curtin (1985), a posterior staphyloma—or *ectasia*—is visualized as a tessellation and pallor of a fundus area around—or to one side of—the optic disk. Although the borders of the ectasia may not be discernible, the tessellation and pallor indicate that a staphyloma is present. Curtin has identified five varieties of posterior staphyloma, based on the area of the fundus in which the staphyloma is located. Four of these types of staphylomas are shown diagrammatically in the drawings in Figure 1.11. By far the most common of these is type I staphyloma, which is located at the posterior pole and is evidenced by a horizontally elliptical area of tessellation and pallor encompassing both the optic nerve head and the macular area. The second most common, type II staphyloma, is smaller than type I staphyloma, with the area of tessellation and pallor extending to the optic nerve head but not beyond it. Types III, IV, and V are all relatively uncommon. Type III, the least common, has a small area of tessellation encompassing the optic nerve head but not the macular area; type IV is a nasal, or inverse, staphyloma extending nasally from the optic nerve head; and type V (extremely rare, not shown in Figure 1.11) extends inferiorly from a tilted optic nerve head.

Retinal Hemorrhages

Retinal hemorrhages are small, round, or irregular hemorrhages near (or even at) the macular area, which are thought to involve the choriocapillaris and the lamina vitrea. According to Curtin (1985), if these hemorrhages occur in the macular area, a variable degree of vision loss and metamorphopsia may occur, but otherwise they usually absorb over a period of weeks with little or no aftereffect.

Lacquer Cracks

Lacquer cracks appear as yellow-white lines, usually more or less horizontally oriented, at or near the posterior pole. They have been variously described as representing fissures in the retinal pigment epithelium-lamina vitrea-choriocapillaris complex, originating as mechanical tears in these tissues, or as sclerosed choroidal vessels. Lacquer cracks impart a guarded prognosis for central vision in later life, particularly if they involve the macular area (Curtin, 1985).

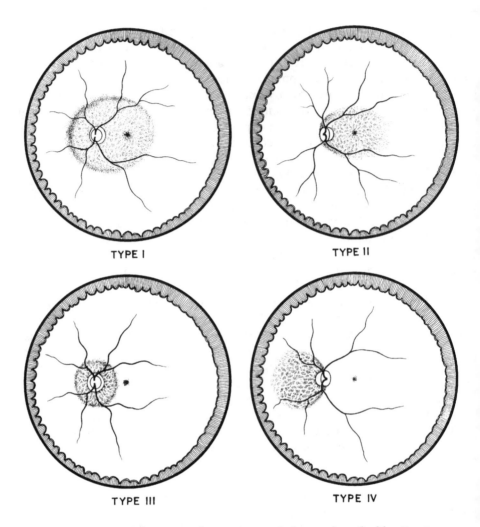

TYPE I

TYPE II

TYPE III

TYPE IV

FIGURE 1.11. Four of the types of posterior staphylomas described by Curtin: type I, the most common, located at the posterior pole and evidenced by a horizontally elliptical area of tessellation and pallor encompassing both the optic nerve head and the macular area; type II, smaller than the type I staphyloma, extending to the optic nerve head but not beyond it; type III, encompassing the optic nerve head but not the macular area; and type IV, a nasal, or inverse, staphyloma extending nasally from the optic nerve head. (Reprinted with permission from BJ Curtin. The Myopias: Basic Science and Clinical Management. Philadelphia: Harper & Row, 1985;302–304.)

Chorioretinal Atrophy

Chorioretinal atrophy appears as small, punched-out, white or yellow irregularly shaped areas, possibly having pigment clumping at their margins, and are usually found in young eyes with advanced staphyloma development. These small atrophic areas tend to increase in size and to coalesce, forming larger lesions which may have clumps of pigment at or near the margins. These changes occur consequent with an increase in the area and depth of the posterior staphyloma, and are due to the occlusion of choroidal end-arteries, signifying a severe loss of choroidal circulation and putting the fundus at risk for the formation of neovascular membranes and subretinal neovascularization (Curtin, 1985).

Subretinal Neovascularization

Once a neovascular membrane has formed beneath the retinal pigment epithelium (between the RPE and the lamina vitrea), the newly formed vessels are prone to leak, in some cases causing extensive hemorrhaging which may produce a central scotoma.

Fuchs' Spot

Sometimes called *Forster-Fuchs' spot*, Fuchs' spot is a round or elliptical pigmented, circumscribed, slightly elevated lesion, usually in the macular area but sometimes in the paramacular area. As described by Blach (1977), it occurs as a result of breaks in Bruch's membrane and the development of a neovascular membrane from the choriocapillaris, giving rise to a hemorrhage which may change color—becoming pigmented—over a period of time. Fuchs' spot initially causes symptoms of metamorphopsia, and may eventually cause a loss of central vision. Although there may be some eventual improvement of vision, the prognosis when Fuchs' spot is present is variously described as "poor" and "guarded."

Peripheral Fundus

Consequent with the axial elongation that is the hallmark of myopia, there occurs an equatorial expansion of the globe: The anterior chamber deepens and the globe becomes larger in its axial, vertical, and transverse dimensions. Curtin (1985) has made the point that even though pathologic changes occurring at the posterior pole can reduce central vision to the level of legal blindness, changes occurring in the retinal periphery pose an even more serious threat to vision because of the possibility of retinal detachment and the complete loss of vision.

A myopic eye is at a greatly increased risk for retinal detachment for a number of reasons, not the least of which is that the prevalence of *vitreous detachment* is much higher in myopic eyes than in emmetropic or hyperopic eyes. Many pathologic changes in the peripheral fundus can be associated with vitreous traction and therefore can lead to vitreous detachment and possibly to retinal detachment. These include white-without-pressure, lattice degeneration, pigmentary degeneration, paving-stone degeneration, and retinal breaks.

White-without-pressure occurs in the form of one or more whitish, circumferentially oriented, flat or slightly elevated areas in the peripheral retina. Curtin (1985) noted that most retinal specialists attribute white-without-pressure to vitreoretinal traction. Curtin has published a graph showing that the prevalence of white-without-pressure increases significantly not only with increasing axial length but with increasing age.

Lattice degeneration is seen as circumferentially oriented, spindle-shaped areas in the peripheral retina, at or beyond the equator. The lesion is pigmented and, as the term indicates, has a latticelike appearance. It consists of a thinning and atrophy of the retina, with liquefaction and detachment of the overlying vitreous. Lattice degeneration indicates an increased risk for retinal holes, tears, and detachment (Goss and Eskridge, 1987).

Pigmentary and *paving-stone degeneration*, as the names imply, consist of pigment deposits and circular yellowish-white areas of degeneration in the peripheral retina. Although they are relatively common and are seen in eyes that are not myopic, they have a higher prevalence in myopic eyes. Both of these conditions are considered to be benign, but pigmentary degeneration may be associated with unidentified areas of lattice degeneration.

Retinal breaks—holes and tears—can be seen in nonmyopic eyes, but have a higher prevalence in myopic eyes. Holes differ from tears in that the holes are round, as the term indicates, whereas tears are usually horseshoe-shaped, with the limbs of the horseshoe aiming peripherally. Retinal tears often occur as a result of traction, and may cause symptoms such as photopsia, vitreous floaters, and smoky vision (Curtin, 1985).

Vitreous Detachment

As we recall from our study of ocular anatomy, the vitreous is attached anteriorly at the vitreous base and posteriorly at the optic nerve head. In myopic eyes, the vitreous gradually *liquefies*, and this liquefaction is, of course, responsible for the fact that myopes—even low and moderate myopes—complain of seeing spots and wiggly "bacteria-shaped" objects in the presence of a bright, uniform background.

When the vitreous detaches, the detachment characteristically occurs at the optic nerve head and is called *posterior detachment and collapse.* Figure 1.12 shows a posterior vitreous collapse, but the vitreous remains attached at the optic nerve head. At the moment of the detachment, the patient sees a *temporal arc of flashes.* These sparklike flashes occur in the temporal field because of the sudden traction—caused by movement of the vitreous body—which occurs on the nasal side of the still-attached vitre-

FIGURE 1.12. Posterior vitreous collapse. Note that the retina remains attached in the area of the optic nerve head. (Reprinted with permission from BJ Curtin. The Myopias: Basic Science and Clinical Management. Philadelphia: Harper & Row, 1985.)

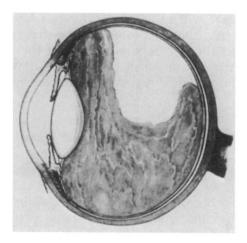

ous base. During the next 24 hours or longer, the patient may repeatedly see the temporal flashes that occur as a result of eye movements—and they can even awake the sleeping patient, apparently due to the rapid eye movements that occur during dreaming. Other, equally disturbing, symptoms may be the visualization of a black ring that tends to move around in the visual field and the perception of a myriad of black dots caused by tiny hemorrhages. The black ring is an image of the pigmented ring resulting from the detachment.

Because vitreous detachment can lead to retinal detachment—concurrently or within several days—it is a *true ophthalmic emergency.* Symptoms of suddenly occurring flashes or a wiggly black ring require an immediate dilated fundus examination and referral for a second opinion.

Retinal Detachment

Retinal detachment in a myopic eye—often referred to as *rhegmatogenous* retinal detachment—is a disorder in which the sensory retina separates from the retinal pigment epithelium, leaving the pigment epithelium attached to the choroid. It occurs as a result of a discontinuity of the retina related to retinal breaks, lattice degeneration, or retinal dialysis (a tearing away of the anterior retina at the ora serrata).

The probability of the occurrence of a retinal detachment is greatest within the first week after a vitreous detachment. If a retinal detachment occurs simultaneously with a vitreous detachment, the symptoms will obviously be those of both conditions. But if a retinal detachment occurs subsequent to a vitreous attachment (which in some cases may not have been reported by the patient), the symptoms will depend on the location of the retinal detachment. The classic symptom of a "curtain in front of the eye" will be present if the detachment involves the macular area; otherwise, the symptoms will be that of a positive scotoma. The patient is likely to "see something" in the visual field that moves away when attempts are made to fixate on it. Such a complaint obviously warrants an immediate visual field evaluation and a dilated fundus examination.

Case Report

Following is a personal case report of one of the authors (TG): Spherical equivalent refractive error for the right eye is –9.50 D; left eye, –4.75 D. In 1981, the patient experienced a suddenly occurring cascade of tiny flashes in the temporal field of the right eye, with no apparent loss of central acuity but with the appearance of a wiggly oval ring. Within the next hour, he had undergone binocular indirect ophthalmoscopy by optometric and ophthalmologic clinic faculty members at the University of Houston College of Optometry, who agreed that there was a posterior vitreous detachment and collapse, but there was no indication of a retinal detachment. During the following days, the temporal flashes occurred several times with extreme eye movements, and the pigmented ring gradually dispersed with no further problems.

Twelve years later, in October 1993, the patient awoke with the realization that he was again seeing a cascade of tiny flashes, but this time in the temporal field of the left eye. Driving to the optometry clinic that morning, he repeatedly saw numerous flocks of birds just above the horizon, which was not unusual in southern Indiana, but it soon became obvious that these "birds" were entoptic phenomena. Binocular indirect ophthalmoscopy, performed at the Indiana University School of Optometry, indicated a vitreous detachment in the left eye with no indication of a retinal detachment. Five days later, however, when on duty in the contact lens clinic, the patient noticed an unidentified object in the nasal visual field of the left eye. Performing confrontations on himself, he found that the positive scotoma was located about as far nasally as the blind spot was temporally—approximately 15 degrees from fixation and somewhat inferior. This field loss was confirmed by a visual field examination by an otherwise idle student clinician, and dilated fundus examinations by several clinic faculty members, including the clinic director, revealed a detachment in the superior temporal retina with no foveal involvement. Thanks to the kindness of a clinic faculty member, the patient was driven to the emergency room of an Indianapolis hospital, where he was met, by prearrangement, by a retinal surgeon who immediately examined him and performed reattachment surgery the next morning. The surgery was highly successful. Unfortunately for most patients who have retinal detachments, the detachment does not occur while at an optometry clinic.

Ocular Morbidity Due to Myopia

Myopia is not only an inconvenience due to the need for glasses or contact lenses, but is also associated with a high level of ocular morbidity. Information concerning the role of myopia as a cause of blindness has been reported by Sorsby (1966, 1972), Perkins (1979), and other authors.

Blind Registrations

Sorsby's reports (1966, 1972) were based on blind registrations in England and Wales, on the basis of bilateral blindness due to the same cause in both eyes. In his 1966 report, myopia was listed as the fourth greatest cause of blindness, being responsible for 8.8% of blind registrations as compared with 26.9% for senile macular degeneration, 22.6% for cataract, and 12.6% for glaucoma. Of the 8.8% of blind registrations due to myopia, 8.4% were listed as due to degenerative myopia and 0.4% due to retinal detachment. When blind registrations were tabulated on the basis of the age at the time of registration, for patients ages 50–59 years, myopia was responsible for the highest percentage of blindness, 18.1%, with diabetic retinopathy second at 15.2%.

In Sorsby's 1972 report, which included blind registrations to age 65, myopia was listed as the third greatest cause of blind registrations, being responsible for 14.0% of blindness as compared with 15.7% for diabetic retinopathy and 14.2% for congenital conditions. For blind registrations between ages 50 and 59 years, myopia was the second greatest cause of blindness, responsible for 18.2% as compared with 19.3% for diabetic retinopathy.

Retinal Detachment

In discussing Sorsby's reports, Perkins (1979) made the point that whereas *bilateral* blindness due to retinal detachment is uncommon, thanks to modern surgical techniques, *unilateral* vision loss is inevitable if the macula becomes detached. On the basis of an analysis of data on patients seen at the Retinal Detachment Unit of Moorefield's Eye Hospital in London, Perkins calculated the annual incidence of 1/20,000. The probability of retinal detachment in a given year for various refractive levels is given in Table 1.18. The information in Table 1.18 shows that the probability of a retinal detachment for an eye with a refractive error of more than −10.00 D is 63,636/148, or 436 times greater than for an eye having a refractive error of +5.00 D.

Glaucoma

The possibility of a relationship between myopia and glaucoma is illustrated by the conclusion by Kelly (1981), a retinal surgeon, that myopia and

TABLE 1.18
Probability of Retinal Detachment as a Function of Refractive Error

Refraction	Probability of Detachment
+5.00 D	1/63,636
0 to +4.75 D	1/48,913
0 to –4.75 D	1/6,662
–5.0 to –9.75 D	1/1,335
>–10.00 D	1/148

Source: Data from ES Perkins. Morbidity from myopia. Sight Sav Rev 1979;(Spring, 49):11–19.

chronic glaucoma are both due to a rise in IOP. After citing data showing that IOP of myopic eyes was found to increase by 1.5 mm Hg when measured in the morning, Kelly suggested that juvenile myopia should be called *expansion glaucoma*. He also suggested that because the eye of an adult is not able to expand, chronic glaucoma in adults should be called *nonexpansion glaucoma*.

Perkins (1979) provided calculations of the probability of glaucoma as related to refractive error on the basis of a data resulting from a glaucoma survey carried out in Bedford, England. Assuming the annual incidence of glaucoma to be 1%, he concluded that open-angle glaucoma is twice as likely to occur in a myopic eye as in an emmetropic eye, and five times as likely as in a hyperopic eye.

Cataract

Perkins (1979) cited Moorefield's Hospital data showing that for a period of 1 year the median refractive error of eyes undergoing cataract surgery was –3.75 D, "with approximately equal distribution on either side of this figure." He went on to say that "the preponderance of myopic refractions can in part be due to an increased refractive power of the cataractous lens." Apparently, the Moorefield's data did not include refractive data *before* cataract development. It is a common clinical finding that many eyes that become myopic due to nuclear sclerosis were hyperopic or emmetropic before the cataract developed.

☼ CLINICAL PEARL

The content of this chapter includes the optics of the myopic eye, the prevalence of myopia and factors associated with variation in prevalence, classification of myopia, risk factors for myopia, typical patterns and rates of myopia progression, factors that affect rates of myopia progression, ocular optical component changes in myopia progression, ocular pathologic changes associated with myopia, and ocular morbidity in myopia. It will be helpful for the reader to keep this information in mind as a background for assessing theories of myopia etiology, for the decision-making process in lens prescribing, for the development and application of myopia control and myopia reduction methods, and for effective communication with patients and other professionals.

References

Abdalla MI, Hamdi M. Applanation ocular tension in myopia and emmetropia. Br J Ophthalmol 1970;54:122–125.

Adams AJ, Baldwin WR, Biederman I, et al. Myopia: Prevalence and Progression. Washington: National Academy Press, 1989;19–21, 26–33, 58–59, 72–84.

Angle J, Wissman DA. The epidemiology of myopia. Am J Epidemiol 1980;111: 220–228.

Araki M. Studies on refractive components of human eye by means of ultrasonic echogram. Report III: the correlation of among refractive components. Acta Soc Ophthalmol Jpn 1962;66:128–147.

Ashton GC. Segregation analysis of ocular refraction and myopia. Hum Hered 1985;35:232–239.

Baldwin WR. Corneal curvature changes in high myopia vs. corneal curvature changes in low myopia. Am J Optom Arch Am Acad Optom 1962;39:349–355.

Baldwin WR, West D, Jolley J, Reid W. Effects of contact lenses on refractive, corneal, and axial length changes in young myopes. Am J Optom Arch Am Acad Optom 1969;46:903–911.

Blach RK. Degenerative Myopia. In Krill's Hereditary Retinal and Choroidal Diseases. Hagerstown, MD: Harper & Row, 1977.

Blum HL, Peters HB, Bettman JW. Vision Screening for Elementary Schools—The Orinda Study. Berkeley, CA: University of California Press, 1959.

Borish IM. Clinical Refraction (3rd ed). Chicago: Professional Press, 1970;5–114.

Bücklers M. Changes in refraction during life. Br J Ophthalmol 1953;37:587–592.

Bullimore MA, Gilmartin B, Royston JM. Steady-state accommodation and ocular biometry in late-onset myopia. Doc Ophthalmol 1992;80:143–155.

Carpel EE, Engstrom PF. The normal cup-disk ratio. Am J Ophthalmol 1981;91:588.

Cook RC, Glasscock RE. Refractive and ocular findings in the newborn. Am J Ophthalmol 1951;34:1407–1413.

Curtin BJ. The Myopias: Basic Science and Clinical Management. Philadelphia: Harper & Row, 1985;17–26, 120–127, 169–175, 237–400.

Drobe B, de Saint-André R. The pre-myopic syndrome. Ophthal Physiol Opt 1995;15:375–378.

Dunphy EB, Stoll MR, King SH. Myopia among American male graduate students. Am J Ophthalmol 1968;65:518–521.

Edwards MH. A Longitudinal Study of the Development of Myopia in Chinese Children: A Life Table Treatment. In T Tokoro (ed), Myopia Updates—Proceedings of the 6th International Conference on Myopia. Tokyo: Springer-Verlag, 1998;48–52.

Edwards MH, Brown B. Intraocular pressure in a selected sample of myopic and non–myopic Chinese children. Optom Vis Sci 1993;70:15–17.

Edwards MH, Brown B. IOP in myopic children: the relationship between increases in IOP and the development of myopia. Ophthal Physiol Opt 1996;16:243–246.

Ehrlich DL, Braddick OJ, Atkinson J, et al. Infant emmetropization: longitudinal changes in refraction components from nine to twenty months of age. Optom Vis Sci 1997;74:822–843.

Erickson P. Mathematical model for predicting dioptric effects of optical parameter changes in the eye. Am J Optom Physiol Opt 1977;54:226–233.

Erickson P. Complete ocular component analysis by vergence contribution. Am J Optom Physiol Opt 1984;61:469–472.

Erickson P. Optical Components Contributing to Refractive Anomalies. In T Grosvenor, MC Flom (eds), Refractive Anomalies: Research and Clinical Applications. Boston: Butterworth–Heinemann, 1991.

Fledelius HC. Changes in eye refraction and eye size during adolescence—with special reference to the influence of low birth weight. In HC Fledelius, PH Alsbirk, E Goldschmidt (eds), Third International Conference on Myopia. Doc Ophthalmol Proc 1981;28:63–69.

Fledelius HC. Is myopia getting more frequent? A cross-sectional study of 1416 Danes aged 16 years +. Acta Ophthalmol 1983;61:545–559.

Fletcher MC, Brandon S. Myopia of prematurity. Am J Ophthalmol 1955;40:474–481.

Francois J, Goes F. Oculometry of progressive myopia. Bibl Ophthalmol 1975;83:277–282.

Fulk GW, Cyert LA. Can bifocals slow myopia progression? J Am Optom Assoc 1996;67:749–754.

Fulk GW, Goss DA, Christensen MT, et al. Optic nerve crescents and refractive error. Optom Vis Sci 1992;69:208–213.

Garner LF, Yap M, Scott R. Crystalline lens power in myopia. Optom Vis Sci 1992;69:863–865.

Garner LF, Meng CK, Grosvenor TP, Mohidin N. Ocular dimensions and refractive power in Malay and Melanesian children. Ophthal Physiol Opt 1990;10:234–238.

Goldschmidt E. On the etiology of myopia—an epidemiological study. Acta Ophthalmol 1968;98(Suppl):1–172.

Goldschmidt E. Refraction in the newborn. Acta Ophthalmol 1969;47:570–578.

Goss DA. Overcorrection as a means of slowing myopia progression. Am J Optom Physiol Opt 1984;61:85–93.

Goss DA. Refractive status and premature birth. Optom Monthly 1985;76:109–111.

Goss DA. Linearity of refractive change with age in childhood myopia progression. Am J Optom Physiol Opt 1987;64:775–780.

Goss DA. Variables related to the rate of childhood myopia progression. Optom Vis Sci 1990;67:631–636.

Goss DA. Clinical accommodation and heterophoria findings preceding juvenile onset of myopia. Optom Vis Sci 1991a;68:110–116.

Goss DA. Childhood Myopia. In T Grosvenor, MC Flom (eds), Refractive Anomalies: Research and Clinical Applications. Boston: Butterworth–Heinemann, 1991b.

Goss DA. Effect of spectacle correction on the progression of myopia in children—a literature review. J Am Optom Assoc 1994;65:117–128.

Goss DA, Cox VD. Trends in the change of clinical refractive error in myopes. J Am Optom Assoc 1985;56:608–613.

Goss DA, Cox VD, Herrin-Lawson GA, et al. Refractive error, axial length, and height as a function of age in young myopes. Optom Vis Sci 1990;67:332–338.

Goss DA, Erickson P. Meridional corneal components of myopia progression in young adults and children. Am J Optom Physiol Opt 1987;64:475–481.

Goss DA, Erickson P. Effects of changes in anterior chamber depth on refractive error in the human eye. Clin Vis Sci 1990;5:197–201.

Goss DA, Eskridge JB. Myopia. In JF Amos (ed), Diagnosis and Management in Vision Care. Boston: Butterworths, 1987.

Goss DA, Jackson TW. Clinical findings before the onset of myopia in youth. 1. Ocular optical components. Optom Vis Sci 1995;72:870–878.

Goss DA, Jackson TW. Clinical findings before the onset of myopia in youth. 2. Zone of clear single binocular vision. Optom Vis Sci 1996a;73:263–268.

Goss DA, Jackson TW. Clinical findings before the onset of myopia in youth. 3. Heterophoria. Optom Vis Sci 1996b;73:269–278.

Goss DA, Jackson TW. Clinical findings before the onset of myopia in youth. 4. Parental history of myopia. Optom Vis Sci 1996c;73:279–282.

Goss DA, Caffey TW. Clinical findings before the onset of myopia in youth. 5. Intraocular pressure. Submitted manuscript.

Goss DA, Rainey BB. Relation of childhood myopia progression rates to time of year. J Am Optom Assoc 1998;69:262–266.

Goss DA, Shewey WB. Rates of childhood myopia progression as a function of type of astigmatism. Clin Exp Optom 1990;73:159–163.

Goss DA, Wickham MG. Retinal–image mediated ocular growth as a mechanism for juvenile onset myopia and for emmetropization—a literature review. Doc Ophthalmol 1995;90:341–375.

Goss DA, Winkler RL. Progression of myopia in youth: age of cessation. Am J Optom Physiol Opt 1983;60:651–658.

Goss DA, Erickson P, Cox VD. Prevalence and pattern of adult myopia progression in a general optometric practice. Am J Optom Physiol Opt 1985;62:470–477.

Goss DA, VanVeen HG, Rainey BB, Feng B. Ocular components measured by keratometry, phakometry, and ultrasonography in emmetropic and myopic optometry students. Optom Vis Sci 1997;74:489–495.

Greene PR. Mechanical Considerations in Myopia. In T Grosvenor, MC Flom (eds), Refractive Anomalies: Research and Clinical Applications. Boston: Butterworth–Heinemann, 1991.

Grosvenor T. A longitudinal study of refractive changes between ages 20 and 40. Part 3: Statistical analysis. Optom Monthly 1977;68:455–457.

Grosvenor T. A review and a suggested classification system for myopia on the basis of age-related prevalence and age of onset. Am J Optom Physiol Opt 1987;64:545–554.

Grosvenor T. Refractive component changes in adult-onset myopia: evidence from five studies. Clin Exp Optom 1994;77:196–205.

Grosvenor T. Primary Care Optometry: Anomalies of Refraction and Binocular Vision (3rd ed). Boston: Butterworth–Heinemann, 1996;37–38, 45–48.

Grosvenor T, Goss DA. Role of the cornea in emmetropia and myopia. Optom Vis Sci 1998;75:132–145.

Grosvenor T, Scott R. Comparison of refractive components of youth-onset and early adult–onset myopia. Optom Vis Sci 1991;68:204–209.

Grosvenor T, Scott R. Three year changes in refraction and its components in youth-onset and early adult–onset myopia. Optom Vis Sci 1993;70:677–683.

Grosvenor T, Scott R. Role of the axial length/corneal radius ratio in determining the refractive state of the eye. Optom Vis Sci 1994;71:573–579.

Grosvenor T, Perrigin DM, Perrigin J, Maslovitz B. Houston myopia control study: a randomized clinical trial. Part II. Final report by the patient care team. Am J Optom Physiol Opt 1987;64:482–498.

Grosvenor T, Perrigin D, Perrigin J, Quintero S. Rigid gas permeable contact lenses for myopia control: effects of discontinuation of lens wear. Optom Vis Sci 1991;68:385–389.

Gwiazda J, Thorn F, Bauer J, Held R. Emmetropization and the progression of manifest refraction in children followed from infancy to puberty. Clin Vis Sci 1993;8:337–344.

Hirai H, Saishin M, Yamamoto K. Longitudinal and Cross-Sectional Study of Refractive Changes in Pupils from 3 to 17 Years of Age. In T Tokoro (ed), Myopia Updates—Proceedings of the 6th International Conference on Myopia. Tokyo: Springer-Verlag, 1998;81–84.

Hirsch MJ. The changes in refraction between the ages of 5 and 14—theoretical and practical considerations. Am J Optom Arch Am Acad Optom 1952;29: 445–459.

Hirsch MJ. Changes in refractive state after the age of 45. Am J Optom Arch Am Acad Optom 1958;35:229–237.

Hirsch MJ. Predictability of refraction at age 14 on the basis of testing at age 6—interim report from the Ojai longitudinal study of refraction. Am J Optom Arch Am Acad Optom 1964;41:567–573.

Ingram RM, Barr A. Changes in refraction between the ages of 1 and 3 1/2 years. Br J Ophthalmol 1979;63:339–342.

Jain IS, Jain S, Mohan K. The epidemiology of high myopia—changing trends. Indian J Ophthalmol 1983;31:723–728.

Jensen H. Myopia Progression in Young School Children. A Prospective Study of Myopia Progression and the Effect of a Trial with Bifocal Lenses and Beta Blocker Eye Drops. Copenhagen: Scriptor, 1991.

Jensen H. Myopia progression in young school children and intraocular pressure. Doc Ophthalmol 1992;82:249–255.

Keller JT. A comparison of the refractive status of myopic children and their parents. Am J Optom Arch Am Acad Optom 1973;50:206–211.

Kelly TS. Myopia or Expansion Glaucoma. In Doc Ophthalmol Proc Series 28; Third Annual Conference on Myopia 1980. The Hague: Dr. Junk, 1981.

Kempf GA, Collins SD, Jarman BL. Refractive Errors in the Eyes of Children as

Determined by Retinoscopic Examination with a Cycloplegic, Public Health Bulletin No. 182. Washington, DC: U.S. Government Printing Office, 1928.

Kent PR. Acquired myopia of maturity. Am J Optom Arch Am Acad Optom 1963;40:247–256.

Ko LS. The problem of myopia in Taiwan. J Korean Ophthalmol Soc 1984;25:591–604.

Krause U, Krause K, Rantakillio P. Sex difference in refractive errors. Acta Ophthalmol 1982;60:917–924.

Kronfeld PC. The early ophthalmoscopic diagnosis of glaucoma. J Am Optom Assoc 1951;23:156–159.

Laatikainen L, Erkkila H. Refractive errors and other ocular findings in school children. Acta Ophthalmol 1980;58:129–136.

Lecaillon-Thibon B. Long-Term Follow-Up Studies of Myopia. In HC Fledelius, PH Alsbirk, E Goldschmidt (eds), Third International Conference on Myopia. Doc Ophthalmol Proc 1981;28:29–32.

Lin LL, Chen CJ, Hung PT, Ko LS. Nation-wide survey of myopia among school-children in Taiwan, 1986. Acta Ophthalmol Suppl 1988;185:29–33.

Lowrey GH. Growth and Development of Children (7th ed). Chicago: Yearbook, 1978;84–85.

Mäntyjärvi M. Incidence of myopia in a population of Finnish school children. Acta Ophthalmol 1983;61:417–423.

Mäntyjärvi MI. Change of refraction in schoolchildren. Arch Ophthalmol 1985a; 103:790–792.

Mäntyjärvi MI. Predicting of myopia progression in school children. J Pediatr Ophthalmol Strab 1985b;22:71–75.

Matsuo C. Studies on spectacles correcting corneal astigmatism for the prevention of progress in myopia. Report III. On the change in ocular refraction under the wearing of spectacles correcting corneal astigmatism. Acta Soc Ophthalmol Jpn 1965;69:165–180.

McBrien NA, Adams DW. A longitudinal investigation of adult-onset and adult-progression of myopia in an occupational group—refractive and biometric findings. Invest Ophthalmol Vis Sci 1997;38:321–333.

McBrien NA, Millodot M. A biometric investigation of late-onset myopic eyes. Acta Ophthalmol 1987;65:461–468.

Mohindra I, Held R. Refraction in Humans from Birth to Five Years. In HC Fledelius, PH Alsbirk, E Goldschmidt (eds), Third International Conference on Myopia. Doc Ophthalmol Proc 1981;28:19–27.

Morgan MW. Analysis of clinical data. Am J Optom Arch Am Acad Optom 1944; 21:477–491.

Mutti DO, Zadnik K. The utility of three predictors of childhood: a Bayesian analysis. Vis Res 1995;35:1345–1352.

O'Neal MR, Connon TR. Refractive error change at the United States Air Force Academy Class of 1985. Am J Optom Physiol Opt 1987;64:344–354.

Ohno S. An analytical study on correlation of refractivity to ocular axial length in adolescents viewed by means of roentgen-vision. Acta Soc Ophthalmol Jpn 1956;60:460–481.

Ong E, Ciuffreda KJ. Accommodation, Nearwork and Myopia. Santa Ana, CA: Optometric Extension Program, 1997.

Otsuka J. Research on the etiology and treatment of myopia. Acta Soc Ophthalmol Jpn 1967;71(Suppl):1–212.

Paritsis N, Sarafidou E, Koliopoulas J, Trichopoulos D. Epidemiologic research on the role of studying and urban environment in the development of myopia during school-age years. Ann Ophthalmol 1983;15:1061–1065.

Pärssinen O. Astigmatism and school myopia. Acta Ophthalmol 1991;69:786–790.

Pärssinen O, Hemminki E, Klemetti A. Effect of spectacle use and accommodation on myopic progression: final results of a three-year randomised clinical trial among schoolchildren. Br J Ophthalmol 1989;73:547–551.

Paul L. Untersuchungen ber der erbliche Entstehung der Kurzichtigkeit. I. Mitteilung. von Graefes Arch Ophthalmol 1938;139:378–402.

Perkins ES. Morbidity from myopia. Sight Sav Rev 1979;(Spring, 49):11–19.

Perkins ES. Myopia and Scleral Stress. In Doc Ophthalmol Proc Series 28; Third Annual Conference on Myopia 1980. The Hague: Dr. Junk, 1981.

Pruett RC. Progressive myopia and intraocular pressure: what is the linkage? A literature review. Acta Ophthalmol Suppl 1988;185:117–127.

Quinn GE, Berlin JA, Young TL, et al. Association of intraocular pressure and myopia in children. Ophthalmology 1995;102:180–185.

Rajan U, Saw S-M, Lau C, et al. Prevalence of Myopia in Schoolchildren and Risk Factors for its Progression. In T Tokoro (ed), Myopia Updates—Proceedings of the 6th International Conference on Myopia. Tokyo: Springer-Verlag, 1998; 69–80.

Richler A, Bear JC. The distribution of refraction in three isolated communities in Western Newfoundland. Am J Optom Physiol Opt 1980;57:861–871.

Roberts WL, Banford RD. Evaluation of Bifocal Correction Technique in Juvenile Myopia. OD Thesis, Massachusetts College of Optometry, Boston, 1963.

Roberts WL, Banford RD. Evaluation of bifocal correction technique in juvenile myopia. Optom Weekly 1967;58(38):25–28, 31; 58(39):21–30; 58(40):23–28; 58(41):27–34; 58(43):19–24, 26.

Rosenberg T, Goldschmidt E. The Onset and Progression of Myopia in Danish School Children. In HC Fledelius, PH Alsbirk, E Goldschmidt (eds), Third International Conference on Myopia. Doc Ophthalmol Proc 1981;28:33–39.

Rosner M, Belkin M. Intelligence, education, and myopia in males. Arch Ophthalmol 1987;105:1508–1511.

Scharf J, Zonis S. Zeltzer M. Refraction in Israeli premature babies. J Pediatr Ophthalmol 1975;12:193–196.

Scott R, Grosvenor T. A structural model for emmetropic and myopic eyes. Ophthal Physiol Opt 1993;13:41–47.

Septon RD. Myopia among optometry students. Am J Optom Physiol Opt 1984;61: 745–751.

Sheridan M. The crystalline lens in myopia. Optician 1955;129:447–450, 456.

Shlaifer A. A Synopsis of Glaucoma for Optometrists. Minneapolis: Burgess, 1959.

Sorsby A. The Incidence of Blindness in England and Wales, 1948–1962. London: Her Majesty's Stationery Office, 1966.

Sorsby A. The Incidence of Blindness in England and Wales, 1963–1968. London: Her Majesty's Stationery Office, 1972.

Sorsby A, Benjamin B, Davey JB, et al. Emmetropia and Its Aberrations. Medical Research Council Special Report Series no. 293. London: Her Majesty's Stationery Office, 1957.

Sorsby A, Leary GA. A Longitudinal Study of Refraction and Its Components During Growth. Medical Research Council Special Report Series no. 309. London: Her Majesty's Stationery Office, 1970.

Sorsby A, Leary GA, Richards MJ. Correlation ametropia and component ametropia. Vis Res 1962;2:309–313.

Sperduto RD, Seigel D, Roberts J, Rowland M. Prevalence of myopia in the United States. Arch Ophthalmol 1983;101:405–407.

Stenstrom S. Investigation of the variation and correlation of the optical elements of human eyes. Part III. Woolf D, translator. Am J Optom Arch Am Acad Optom 1948a;25:340–350.

Stenstrom S. Investigation of the variation and correlation of the optical elements of human eyes. Part IV. Woolf D, translator. Am J Optom Arch Am Acad Optom 1948b;25:438–449.

Sutton MR, Ditmars DL. Vision problems at West Point. J Am Optom Assoc 1970;41:263–265.

Tokoro T, Kabe S. Relations between changes in the ocular refraction and refractive components and the development of the myopia. Acta Soc Ophthalmol Jpn 1964a;68:1240–1253.

Tokoro T, Kabe S. Treatment of myopia and the changes in optical components. Report I. Topical application of Neosynephrine and tropicamide. Acta Soc Ophthalmol Jpn 1964b;68:1958–1961.

Tokoro T, Kabe S. Treatment of myopia and the changes in optical components. Report II. Full or under-correction of myopia by glasses. Acta Soc Ophthalmol Jpn 1965;69:140–144.

Tomlinson A, Phillips CI. Applanation tension and axial length of the eyeball. Br J Ophthalmol 1970;54:548–553.

Tsai C-B, Lin LL-K, Shih Y-F, Hung P-T. Prevalence and Patterns of Myopic Progression among Schoolchildren: Eight Year Longitudinal Study. In T Tokoro (ed), Myopia Updates—Proceedings of the 6th International Conference on Myopia. Tokyo: Springer-Verlag, 1998;67.

U.S. Department of Health, Education, and Welfare. Refraction Status and Motility Defects of Persons 4–74 Years, United States, 1971–72, HEW Publication No. (PHS) 78-1654. Hyattsville, MD: U.S. Department of Health, Education, and Welfare, 1978.

van Alphen GWHM. On emmetropia and ametropia. Ophthalmologica 1961;142(Suppl):1–92.

Wold KC. Hereditary myopia. Arch Ophthalmol 1949;42:225–237.

Yamamoto M, Tatsugami H, Bun J. A follow-up study of refractive error in premature infants. Jpn J Ophthalmol 1979;23:435–443.

Young FA. The development and control of myopia in human and subhuman primates. Contacto 1975;19:16–31.

Young FA. The nature and control of myopia. J Am Optom Assoc 1977;48:451–457.

Young FA, Leary GA. Accommodation and Vitreous Chamber Pressure: A Proposed Mechanism for Myopia. In T Grosvenor, MC Flom (eds), Refractive Anomalies: Research and Clinical Applications. Boston: Butterworth–Heinemann, 1991.

Young FA, Beattie RJ, Newby FJ, Swindal MT. The Pullman study—a visual survey of Pullman schoolchildren. Part II. Am J Optom Arch Am Acad Optom 1954;31:192–203.

Zadnik K, Mutti DO. Refractive error changes in law students. Am J Optom Physiol Opt 1987;64:558–561.

Zadnik K, Mutti DO, Friedman NE, Adams AJ. Initial cross-sectional results from the Orinda longitudinal study of myopia. Optom Vis Sci 1993;70:750–758.

Zadnik K, Satariano WA, Mutti DO, et al. The effect of parental history of myopia on children's eye size. J Am Med Assoc 1994;271:1323–1327.

CHAPTER 2

Etiology of Myopia

Myopia causation is the topic of hundreds of scientific papers and numerous scholarly treatises. It is a fascinating topic in and of itself, and it shows the importance of the contributions and interaction of clinical scientists, observant clinical practitioners, and basic scientists. However, for the purposes of examining the clinical management of myopia, we can address the etiology of myopia by asking three questions: (1) Is myopia the result of inheritance, environmental factors, or both? (2) If the environment plays a role in myopia development, can we identify likely physiologic mechanisms? (3) Given the likely environmental contributors to myopia development and their physiologic mechanisms, can we identify potential methods of myopia control or myopia prevention? We present a brief overview of some studies that may shed some light on these questions.

Is Myopia the Result of Inheritance, Environmental Factors, or Both?

One potential approach to this question is to examine whether there is familial resemblance in myopia. Several studies have reported prevalence of myopia as a function of parental history of myopia. These studies are summarized in Table 1.11, and show that parental history of myopia is a risk factor for myopia development. The limitation of these results is that common family lifestyle as well as inheritance may be part of that risk.

The mode of transmission of a condition determined by a single gene can often be discerned by pedigree studies. A review of pedigree studies on myopia concluded that a consistent mode of transmission of myopia has not been identified (Goss et al., 1988). Potential explanations are as follows:

1. Refractive error is a continuous variable rather than a discrete variable. Pedigree studies are more appropriate in studying discrete variables, such as blood type, where categories are obvious, as opposed to

most numerical data which, like refractive error, can be expressed on a continuum, with categories being established only by setting arbitrary numerical limits.

2. Refractive error is affected by multiple genes (polygenic) rather than one gene.
3. Environment may affect refractive development.

Bear (1991) noted that the high peak of the distribution of refractive errors near emmetropia and the fact that very slight anatomic changes can result in significant changes in refractive error indicate that the control of ocular development must be very precise. As a consequence, it is likely that multiple genes contribute to refractive development and that

> genes or environmental factors that do not greatly derange other aspects of development might confer a large refractive error; and commonly occurring environmental influences, though having only a slight influence on ocular development, might nonetheless contribute substantially to population variation in refractive error. (Bear, 1991, p. 58)

He further observed that, because slight anatomic changes in the eye can result in significant refractive errors, it is extremely difficult to determine the exact proportion of variation in refractive error that can be ascribed to particular genetic or environmental influences.

One approach to the question of the relative importance of inheritance and environment is the use of the statistic heritability. Heritability is a statistic that estimates the proportion of phenotypic variation due to polygenic variation, the remainder being assumed to be due to variation in environment and random variation in developmental events. It can be calculated based either on the correlation of parent-offspring data or on the comparison of correlations of monozygous and dizygous twin data. Table 2.1 summarizes the results of various heritability studies on refractive error. The results vary from study to study and from population to popula-

TABLE 2.1
Heritabilities of Refractive Error from Several Studies

Study	Heritability
Kimura (1965), Japan, twin data	0.81
Sorsby et al. (1966), England, parent-offspring data	0.45
Nakajima et al. (1968), Japan, parent-offspring data	0.42
Nakajima et al. (1968), Japan, twin data	0.71
Young and Leary (1972), northern Alaska, parent-offspring data	0.46
Alsbirk (1979), Greenland, parent-offspring data	0.14
Johnson et al. (1979), Labrador, parent-offspring data	0.00
Goss et al. (1988), twin data of Sorsby et al. (1962), England	0.87

tion, but suggest overall that both inheritance and other factors are important in refractive development.

Another way to address the inheritance/environment question is to determine whether any specific environmental factor can be related to greater myopia prevalence or progression. The environmental factor that is frequently associated with myopia is near work. We do not attempt to discuss all of the very extensive literature on near work and myopia. The many studies relating near work to myopia have been summarized in several reviews (Goldschmidt, 1968; Grosvenor, 1977; Baldwin, 1981; Curtin, 1985; Adams et al., 1989; Bear, 1991; Birnbaum, 1993; Ong and Ciuffreda, 1997). These reviews show that the prevalence of myopia is greater among persons who have occupations requiring near work. As a group, myopes do more reading and nearpoint activities, achieve higher educational status, and are better readers than emmetropes and hyperopes.

A sampling of other papers also shows a relation of near work and myopia. Myopia is less common in populations in which there is no compulsory schooling (Young et al., 1969; Garner et al., 1985; Bear, 1991). A greater amount of time spent on reading and near work has been associated with higher rates of childhood myopia progression (Pärssinen et al., 1989; Pärssinen and Lyyra, 1993). Two studies have found lower childhood myopia progression during the 6 months that include summer vacation than during the other 6 months of the year (Fulk and Cyert, 1996; Goss and Rainey, 1998) (Figure 2.1). Zylbermann et al. (1993) reported that teenage Orthodox Jewish male students, who had considerable near work requirements, had much higher prevalences of myopia (81.3% compared with 27.4% of males in general schools). After reviewing epidemiologic studies in various populations, Bear (1991) concluded, "the association of myopia with formal education is strong, remarkably consistent, and dose-dependent" (p. 65). A National Academy of Sciences working group on myopia prevalence and progression (Adams et al., 1989) drew the succinct conclusion that "Doing near work places one at risk for myopia" (p. 1).

It appears, then, that the answer to our first question is that myopia is influenced by both inheritance and environmental factors. Furthermore, it appears that the environmental element that has the most impact is near work.

Can We Identify Likely Physiologic Mechanisms by Which Near Work Plays a Role in Myopia Development?

Through the years many hypotheses have been proposed for mechanisms by which near work could induce myopia. One hypothesis suggests that sustained accommodation causes increased intraocular pressure in the vitreous chamber, which then causes stretching of the posterior segment and

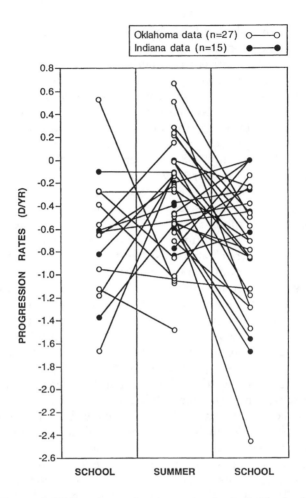

FIGURE 2.1. Rates of childhood myopia progression for individual subjects in the 6 months during the school year and in the 6 months that included the summer vacation. Rates for one "summer period" and one "school-year period" are shown for each subject. For 15 of the subjects, the 6-month school period preceded the 6 months that included the summer period. For 27 subjects, the school period followed the summer period. Although the results are quite variable, most subjects had rates that were less minus during the summer period. Data collected in Oklahoma are represented with solid circles, and data collected in Indiana are represented with open circles. (Data from DA Goss, BB Rainey. Relation of childhood myopia progression rates to time of year. J Am Optom Assoc 1998;69:262–266.)

axial myopia (Young, 1975, 1977, 1981, 1991). This appears to be contradicted by the studies that have found that intraocular pressure measured at the cornea decreases during accommodation (Armaly and Burian, 1958; Armaly and Rubin, 1961; Armaly and Jepson, 1962; Mauger et al., 1984). Young (1991) suggested that a vitreous chamber pressure increase could occur if accommodation caused a pressure gradient between the anterior chamber and the vitreous chamber. Although intraocular pressure has been observed in some studies to be higher in myopes than in hyperopes, work by Edwards and Brown (1996) suggests that intraocular pressure increases after the onset of myopia rather than leading to its onset.

A theory proposed by van Alphen (1961, 1986) states that the eye attempts to adjust axial length to match the refractive power of the eye by allowing or preventing intraocular pressure from stretching the eye longer. He suggested that the ciliary muscle and choroid formed an elastic envelope that resists intraocular pressure and thus limits the stretching of the posterior segment of the eye. In this theory, stimulation of the parasympathetic nervous system (thereby increasing accommodation) would increase the tension in the ciliary muscle and choroid, thus preventing stretch. Myopia results when choroidal tension is insufficient to resist intraocular pressure. One way in which van Alphen suggested that could occur would be in the learning situation where there may be sympathetic stimulation due to the stress of learning leading to relaxation of tension in the ciliary muscle and choroid. He distinguished between close work in general and close work for the purpose of learning, the latter more likely to lead to stress, sympathetic stimulation, decreased choroidal tension, and thus myopia.

Based on engineering principles and calculations, Greene (1980, 1991) suggested that myopia might result from stretch of the posterior sclera induced by a combined influence of the extraocular muscles and pressure within the globe. Greene did not think that the ciliary muscle was strong enough to have a significant mechanical effect on the sclera. He suggested that a mechanical effect on the sclera from near viewing would more likely come from convergence than from accommodation. Ong and Ciuffreda (1997) have given several arguments against the idea that the sclera is mechanically stretched in myopia.

Most attention today centers on a hypothesis that retinal image clarity provides feedback to modulate the rate of posterior segment enlargement. Posterior segment enlargement would accelerate if a point behind the retina were the place at which the best focus would be achieved. That condition would exist for persons with a high lag of accommodation doing near work. Evidence for this theory comes from a variety of research avenues, including laboratory research with animals as well as clinical research. An appealing aspect of this theory is that separate mechanisms do not have to be postulated for myopia and for emmetropization. Myopia development can be viewed as an "emmetropization for near." (See Wallman, 1991; Goss and Zhai, 1994; Goss and Wickham, 1995; Norton and

Siegwart, 1995; Edwards, 1996; Wildsoet, 1997; and Ong and Ciuffreda, 1997, for detailed reviews.)

Emmetropization is a theorized process that guides refractive development toward emmetropia, thus explaining the observation that emmetropia is more common than would be expected by random variation. Various lines of evidence show that emmetropization is a vision dependent phenomenon. Degradation of retinal image quality in several animal species, such as by lid suture or translucent occluders, results in a wide range of refractive errors and a predominance of axial myopia, instead of emmetropia (see reviews by Goss and Criswell, 1981; Criswell and Goss, 1983; Yinon, 1983; Raviola and Wiesel, 1985; Smith, 1991; Edwards, 1996). Conditions in humans that obscure normal retinal imagery, such as lid hemangiomas, ptosis, retrolental fibroplasia associated with retinopathy of prematurity, and vitreous hemorrhage, result in high myopia in infants and children (Robb, 1977; Hoyt et al., 1981; Rabin et al., 1981; Nathan et al., 1985; Miller-Meeks et al., 1990). Axial elongation of the eye has been found to occur in infants and children as a result of eyelid closure, corneal opacification, and congenital cataracts (Hoyt et al., 1981; Gee and Tabbara, 1988; Rasooly and BenEzra, 1988; Kugelberg et al., 1996).

Some of the first evidence for refractive development being modulated by retinal image focus came from work with chickens. Defocus of the retinal image with minus lenses caused acceleration of enlargement of the vitreous chamber and myopia, and plus lenses caused a slowing of axial elongation of the eye and hyperopia (Schaeffel et al., 1988, 1991; Irving et al., 1991). Defocus itself rather than the process of accommodation was found to be responsible for this effect, because axial elongation occurred even though animals were rendered incapable of accommodation by Edinger-Westphal nucleus ablation (Schaeffel et al., 1990).

Defocus was shown to alter refractive development in infant monkeys (Hung et al. 1995). Eleven infant rhesus monkeys were raised wearing lightweight helmets containing lenses. The left lens worn by each monkey was a zero-powered lens. The lens over the right eye was either a +6, +3, 0, –3, or –6 D lens. The helmets were worn for 72–113 days, starting at age 21–32 days. Refractive errors, measured by retinoscopy, ranged from +2.00 to +8.00 D at the beginning of treatment. In most of the monkeys treated with a minus lens, there was more axial elongation and a myopic refractive shift in the treated eye. In the monkeys treated with plus lenses, there was generally less axial elongation and a hyperopic shift in the treated eye. The results, summarized in Figure 2.2, show that the refractive development of primates may be affected by defocus of retinal imagery.

Next, we can ask how such research findings relate to human myopia. If a minus lens is placed before an eye, the focal point of ocular imagery is shifted posteriorly. The defocus theory suggests that over some period of time retinal position is altered to better coincide with the focal plane. The focal point of a nearpoint object would be behind the retina if

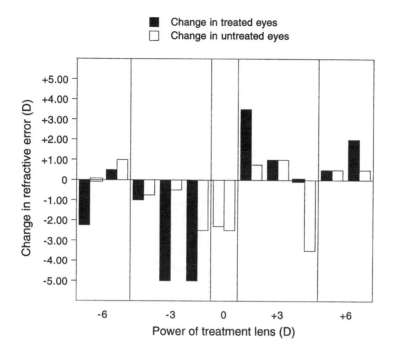

FIGURE 2.2. Changes in refractive error in 11 infant monkeys raised with light-weight helmets containing lenses. The left lens was zero power lens in each monkey. The power of the right lens was –6, –3, 0, +3, or +6 D. (Data from L-F Hung, MLJ Crawford, EL Smith. Spectacle lenses alter eye growth and the refractive status of young monkeys. Nature Med 1995;1:761–765; figure modified from J Wallman, S McFadden. Monkey eyes grow into focus. Nature Med 1995;1:737–739.)

the dioptric accommodative response is less than the dioptric accommodative stimulus. Thus, myopia could result when an individual does a certain amount of near work and has a deficient accommodative response. We have already discussed the evidence that near work is related to myopia. We now turn to the topic of differences in accommodation between myopes and nonmyopes. (See Rosenfield, 1994; Goss and Zhai, 1994; Ong and Ciuffreda, 1997, for reviews.)

McBrien and Millodot (1986) measured accommodative response and slopes of the plot of accommodative response as a function of accommodative stimulus for 40 subjects ages 18–23 years. Accommodative response was measured at accommodative stimulus levels from 0 to 5 D in four refractive groups. Subjects with myopia showed higher lags of accommodation for higher accommodative stimulus levels than emmetropes. Accommodative responses for the 4 and 5 D accommodative stimuli were significantly different between the groups ($p < .05$). The mean slopes for the accommodative response/accommodative stimulus function were 0.87 for myopes with

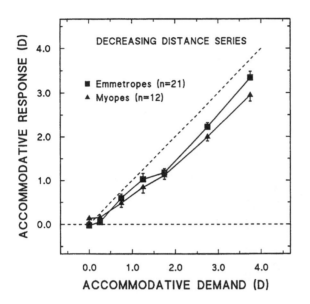

FIGURE 2.3. Accommodative responses in myopic and emmetropic children as a function of accommodative stimulus varied by changes in viewing distance. (Reprinted with permission from J Gwiazda, F Thorn, J Bauer, R Held. Myopic children show insufficient accommodative response to blur. Invest Ophthalmol Vis Sci 1993;34:690–694.)

onset of myopia after age 15 years, 0.88 for myopes with onset of myopia at or before age 13 years, 0.92 for emmetropes, and 0.97 for hyperopes. Slopes had a statistically significant correlation with refractive error ($r = 0.5$, p <.001). Rosenfield and Gilmartin (1990) found lower levels of proximally induced accommodation in early adult–onset myopes than in emmetropes.

Gwiazda et al. (1993) measured accommodative response in 64 children with ages ranging from 5 to 17 years. The mean accommodative response levels for a 33-cm viewing distance were 2.00 D in myopes and 2.22 D in emmetropes. For a 25-cm viewing distance, mean levels were 2.95 D in myopes and 3.34 D in emmetropes. The mean slopes of the accommodative response/accommodative stimulus function were 0.78 in myopic children and 0.88 in emmetropic children, which were significantly different (p <.05). An even greater difference in slope was observed when accommodative stimulus was increased with minus lenses: 0.20 in myopes, as compared with 0.61 in emmetropes. These results are illustrated in Figures 2.3 and 2.4.

Most studies that have compared dark focus of accommodation levels in myopes and emmetropes have found lower dioptric levels in myopes (Maddock et al., 1981; Smith, 1983; Bullimore et al., 1988; Rosner and Rosner, 1989). Overall the studies on accommodation in myopes and emmetropes suggest that accommodation tends to be less in myopes. However, the question of whether the low accommodative response precedes the myopia, or vice versa, remains open (Gwiazda et al., 1995).

Although there are many laboratory and clinical observations consistent with the defocus theory, some limitations of the application of the existing animal model research to human myopia have been noted (Zadnik

FIGURE 2.4. Accommoda-
tive responses in myopic
and emmetropic children
as a function of accom-
modative stimulus varied
by minus lenses while subjects viewed letters at a
distance of 4 m. (Reprinted
with permission from J
Gwiazda, F Thorn, J Bauer,
R Held. Myopic children
show insufficient accom-
modative response to blur.
Invest Ophthalmol Vis Sci
1993;34:690–694.)

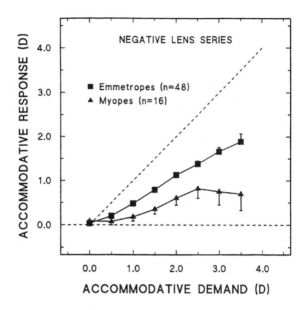

and Mutti, 1998). For example, it would be valuable if future animal studies
used the lower amounts of defocus or contrast reduction, as would occur
with small changes in lag of accommodation, and if the animals were at a
comparable developmental age to school-age children when the onset of
myopia is most common in humans.

In experimentally induced myopia in chickens and monkeys, retinal
biochemistry is affected. Some biochemical agents that affect retinal function can induce myopia, and some can block it (Iuvone et al., 1989; Stone
et al., 1989; Crewther and Crewther, 1990). In chickens, the enlargement
of the vitreous chamber in experimentally induced myopia is due to scleral
growth (Christensen and Wallman, 1991; McBrien et al., 1991; Rada and
Matthews, 1994). Therefore, it appears that in chickens defocus alters retinal activity, which, in turn, modifies scleral growth rate. A similar mechanism may be operative in primates, although it is unclear whether there is
modification of scleral growth rates or whether there may be some form of
scleral remodeling to alter axial length or perhaps scleral remodeling to
make it more likely that intraocular pressure would stretch the posterior
segment (Norton and Siegwart, 1995).

The second question we asked is whether physiologic mechanisms
could be identified by which the environment—specifically near work—
plays a role in myopia development. In the last 25 or 30 years, there have
been two prevailing theories to explain the effect of near work on refractive error. One of these suggests that the process of accommodation some-
how mechanically stretches the sclera. In the formulation of this theory by
Francis Young, increased intraocular pressure causes the scleral stretching.
The other theory is the defocus theory, in which retinal image clarity pro-

vides feedback for refractive development. At the present, there appears to be more support for the defocus theory.

Given the Likely Physiologic Mechanisms of Near Work–Induced Myopia, Can We Identify Potential Methods of Myopia Control or Prevention?

If the process of accommodation plays a role in myopia development, then a strategy for slowing myopia progression (myopia control) or myopia prevention would be to minimize accommodation as much as possible. Higher power plus lens additions (+2.00 to +2.50 D) would be indicated for near work. Recommendations could include not reading continuously for extended periods.

If the defocus theory is correct, then the objective is to maximize retinal image clarity. This could be achieved also by nearpoint plus lens additions, but the powers would not need to be very high. Add powers could be determined by standard means, such as dynamic retinoscopy, relative accommodation findings, amount of esophoria, the gradient accommodative convergence–to–accommodation (AC/A) ratio, and so on. If the human eye is not sensitive to the direction of defocus but rather just the presence of defocus, then both distance and near should be corrected optimally. If the human eye can sense the direction of defocus, then the optimal correction for distance vision would be less important—distance vision could be undercorrected. The prescription of bifocal lenses and progressive addition lenses for myopia control is discussed in Chapter 6. Alternatively, it may be possible to design vision training programs to improve accommodative response and thus decrease the level of defocus. Vision therapy for myopia is discussed in Chapter 5. Recommendations for "visual hygiene" could also be made. For example, because accommodative response decreases as illumination decreases, a recommendation to read under good illumination would be logical. Lag of accommodation increases as viewing distance decreases, so maintaining a minimum reading distance would also be reasonable. Other such visual hygiene principles could be identified.

Conclusion

Based on available studies, we can conclude that both inheritance and environmental factors affect refractive development. The environmental factor that appears to be most important in myopia development is near work. A commonly held theory today is that defocus of the retinal image, such as by a high lag of accommodation during reading, induces accelerated axial elongation of the eye and produces myopia. The defocus theory suggests some reasonable approaches to myopia control and myopia prevention.

References

Adams AJ, Baldwin WR, Biederman I, et al. Myopia: Prevalence and Progression. Washington, DC: National Academy Press, 1989;1–2, 10–22, 58–59.

Alsbirk PH. Refraction in adult West Greenland Eskimos: a population study of spherical refractive errors, including oculometric and familial correlations. Acta Ophthalmologica 1979;57:84–95.

Armaly MF, Burian HM. Changes in the tonogram during accommodation. Arch Ophthalmol 1958;60:60–69.

Armaly MF, Jepson NC. Accommodation and the dynamics of steady-state intraocular pressure. Invest Ophthalmol 1962;1:480–483.

Armaly MF, Rubin ML. Accommodation and applanation tonometry. Arch Ophthalmol 1961;65:415–423.

Baldwin WR. A review of statistical studies of relations between myopia and ethnic, behavioral, and physiological characteristics. Am J Optom Physiol Opt 1981;58:516–527.

Bear JC. Epidemiology and Genetics of Refractive Anomalies. In T Grosvenor, MC Flom (eds), Refractive Anomalies, Research and Clinical Applications. Boston: Butterworth–Heinemann, 1991.

Birnbaum MH. Optometric Management of Nearpoint Vision Disorders. Boston: Butterworth–Heinemann, 1993;12–15.

Bullimore M, Boyd T, Mather HE, Gilmartin B. Near retinoscopy and refractive error. Clin Exp Optom 1988;71:114–118.

Christensen AM, Wallman J. Evidence that increased scleral growth underlies visual deprivation myopia in chicks. Invest Ophthalmol Vis Sci 1991;32:2143–2150.

Crewther DP, Crewther SG. Pharmacological modification of eye growth in normally reared and visually deprived chicks. Curr Eye Res 1990;9:733–740.

Criswell MH, Goss DA. Myopia development in nonhuman primates—a literature review. Am J Optom Physiol Opt 1983;60:250–268.

Curtin BJ. The Myopias: Basic Science and Clinical Management. Philadelphia: Lippincott, 1985;120–129.

Edwards MH. Animal models of myopia—a review. Acta Ophthalmol Scand 1996;74:213–219.

Edwards MH, Brown B. IOP in myopic children: the relationship between increases in IOP and the development of myopia. Ophthal Physiol Opt 1996;16:243–246.

Fulk GW, Cyert LA. Can bifocals slow myopia progression? J Am Optom Assoc 1996;67:749–754.

Garner LF, Kinnear RF, Klinger JD, McKellar MJ. Prevalence of myopia in school children in Vanuatu. Acta Ophthalmol 1985;63:323–326.

Gee SS, Tabbara KF. Increase in ocular axial length in patients with corneal opacification. Ophthalmol 1988;95:1276–1278.

Goldschmidt E. On the etiology of myopia—an epidemiological study. Acta Ophthalmol 1968;98(Suppl):1–172.

Goss DA, Criswell MH. Myopia development in experimental animals—a literature review. Am J Optom Physiol Opt 1981;58:859–869.

Goss DA, Rainey BB. Relation of childhood myopia progression rates to time of year. J Am Optom Assoc 1998;69:262–266.

Goss DA, Wickham MG. Retinal-image mediated ocular growth as a mechanism for juvenile onset myopia and for emmetropization—a literature review. Doc Ophthalmol 1995;90:341–375.

Goss DA, Zhai H. Clinical and laboratory investigations of the relationship of accommodation and convergence function with refractive error—a literature review. Doc Ophthalmol 1994;86:349–380.

Goss DA, Hampton MJ, Wickham MG. Selected review on genetic factors in myopia. J Am Optom Assoc 1988;59:875–884.

Greene PR. Mechanical considerations in myopia: relative effects of accommodation, convergence, intraocular pressure, and the extraocular muscles. Am J Optom Physiol Opt 1980;57:902–914.

Greene PR. Mechanical Considerations in Myopia. In T Grosvenor, MC Flom (eds), Refractive Anomalies, Research and Clinical Applications. Boston: Butterworth–Heinemann, 1991.

Grosvenor T. Are visual anomalies related to reading ability? J Am Optom Assoc 1977;48:510–516.

Gwiazda J, Bauer J, Thorn F, Held R. A dynamic relationship between myopia and blur-driven accommodation in school-aged children. Vis Res 1995;35:1299–1304.

Gwiazda J, Thorn F, Bauer J, Held R. Myopic children show insufficient accommodative response to blur. Invest Ophthalmol Vis Sci 1993;34:690–694.

Hoyt CS, Stone RD, Fromer C, Billson FA. Monocular axial myopia associated with neonatal eyelid closure in human infants. Am J Ophthalmol 1981;91:197–200.

Hung L-F, Crawford MLJ, Smith EL. Spectacle lenses alter eye growth and the refractive status of young monkeys. Nature Med 1995;1:761–765.

Irving EL, Callender MG, Sivak JG. Inducing myopia, hyperopia, and astigmatism. Optom Vis Sci 1991;68:364–368.

Iuvone PM, Tigges M, Fernandes A, Tigges J. Dopamine synthesis and metabolism in rhesus monkey retina: development, aging and the effects of monocular visual deprivation. Vis Neurosci 1989;2:465–471.

Johnson GJ, Matthews A, Perkins ES. Survey of ophthalmic conditions in a Labrador community. I. Refractive errors. Br J Ophthalmol 1979;63:440–448.

Kimura T. Developmental change of the optical components in twins. Acta Soc Ophthalmol Jpn 1965;69:963–969.

Kugelberg U, Zetterström C, Syren-Nordqvist S. Ocular axial length in children with unilateral congenital cataract. Acta Ophthalmol Scand 1996;74:220–223.

Maddock RJ, Millodot M, Leat S, Johnson CA. Accommodation response and refractive error. Invest Ophthalmol Vis Sci 1981;20:387–391.

Mauger RR, Likens CP, Applebaum M. Effects of accommodation and repeated applanation tonometry on intraocular pressure. Am J Optom Physiol Opt 1984;61:28–30.

McBrien NA, Millodot M. The effect of refractive error on the accommodative response gradient. Ophthal Physiol Opt 1986;6:145–149.

McBrien NA, Moghaddam HO, Reeder AP, Moules S. Structural and biochemical changes in the sclera of experimentally myopic eyes. Biochem Soc Trans 1991;19:861–865.

Miller-Meeks MJ, Bennett SR, Keech RV, Blodi CF. Myopia induced by vitreous hemorrhage. Am J Ophthalmol 1990;109:199–203.

Nakajima A, Kimura T, Kitamura K, et al. Studies on the heritability of some metric traits of the eye and the body. Jpn J Human Genet 1968;13:20–39.

Nathan J, Kiely PM, Crewther SG, Crewther DP. Disease associated visual image degradation and spherical refractive errors in children. Am J Optom Physiol Opt 1985;62:680–688.

Norton TT, Siegwart JT Jr. Animal models of emmetropization: matching axial length to the focal plane. J Am Optom Assoc 1995;66:405–414.

Ong E, Ciuffreda KJ. Accommodation, Nearwork and Myopia. Santa Ana, CA: Optometric Extension Program, 1997;76–93.

Pärssinen O, Lyyra AL. Myopia and myopic progression among schoolchildren: a three-year follow-up study. Invest Ophthalmol Vis Sci 1993;34:2794–2802.

Pärssinen O, Hemminki E, Klemetti A. Effect of spectacle use and accommodation on myopic progression: final results of a three-year randomised clinical trial among schoolchildren. Br J Ophthalmol 1989;73:547–551.

Rabin J, Van Sluyters RC, Malach R. Emmetropization: a vision-dependent phenomenon. Invest Ophthalmol Vis Sci 1981;20:561–564.

Rada JA, Matthews AL. Visual deprivation upregulates extracellular matrix synthesis by chick scleral chondrocytes. Invest Ophthalmol Vis Sci 1994;35:2436–2447.

Rasooly R, BenEzra D. Congenital and traumatic cataract—the effect on ocular axial length. Arch Ophthalmol 1988;106:1066–1068.

Raviola E, Wiesel TN. An animal model of myopia. N Engl J Med 1985;312:1609–1615.

Robb RM. Refractive errors associated with hemangiomas of the eyelids and orbit in infancy. Am J Ophthalmol 1977;83:52–58.

Rosenfield M. Accommodation and myopia—are they related? J Behav Optom 1994;5:3–11, 25.

Rosenfield M, Gilmartin B. Effect of target proximity on the open-loop accommodative response. Optom Vis Sci 1990;67:74–79.

Rosner J, Rosner J. Relation between clinically measured tonic accommodation and refractive status in 6- to 14-year-old children. Optom Vis Sci 1989;66:436–439.

Schaeffel F, Howland HC. Properties of the feedback loops controlling eye growth and refractive state in the chicken. Vis Res 1991;31:717–734.

Schaeffel F, Glasser A, Howland HC. Accommodation, refractive error, and eye growth in chickens. Vis Res 1988;28:639–657.

Schaeffel F, Troilo D, Wallman J, Howland HC. Developing eyes that lack accommodation grow to compensate for imposed defocus. Vis Neurosci 1990;4:177–183.

Smith EL III. Experimentally induced refractive anomalies in mammals. In T Grosvenor, MC Flom (eds), Refractive Anomalies, Research and Clinical Applications. Boston: Butterworth–Heinemann, 1991.

Smith G. The accommodative resting states, instrument accommodation and their measurement. Optica Acta 1983;30:347–359.

Sorsby A, Leary GA, Fraser GR. Family studies on ocular refraction and its components. J Med Genet 1966;3:269–273.

Sorsby A, Sheridan M, Leary GA. Refraction and its Components in Twins. Medical Research Council Special Report Series No. 303. London: Her Majesty's Stationery Office, 1962.

Stone RA, Lin T, Laties AM, Iuvone PM. Retinal dopamine and form-deprivation myopia. Proc Nat Acad Sci U S A 1989;86:704–706.

van Alphen GWHM. On emmetropia and ametropia. Ophthalmologica (Basel) 1961;142(Suppl):1–92.

van Alphen GWHM. Choroidal stress and emmetropization. Vis Res 1986; 26:723–734.

Wallman J. Retinal Factors in Myopia and Emmetropization: Clues from Research on Chicks. In T Grosvenor, MC Flom (eds), Refractive Anomalies, Research and Clinical Applications. Boston: Butterworth–Heinemann, 1991.

Wallman J, McFadden S. Monkey eyes grow into focus. Nature Med 1995;1:737–739.

Wildsoet CF. Active emmetropization—evidence for its existence and ramifications for clinical practice. Ophthal Physiol Opt 1997;17:279–290.

Yinon U. Myopia induction in animals following alteration of visual input during development: a review. Curr Eye Res 1983;3:677–690.

Young FA. The development and control of myopia in human and subhuman primates. Contacto 1975;19:16–31.

Young FA. The nature and control of myopia. J Am Optom Assoc 1977;48:451–457.

Young FA. Primate myopia. Am J Optom Physiol Opt 1981;58:560–566.

Young FA. Accommodation and Vitreous Chamber Pressure: A Proposed Mechanism for Myopia. In T Grosvenor, MC Flom (eds), Refractive Anomalies, Research and Clinical Applications. Boston: Butterworth–Heinemann, 1991.

Young FA, Leary GA. The inheritance of ocular components. Am J Optom Arch Am Acad Optom 1972;49:546–555.

Young FA, Leary GA, Baldwin WR, et al. The transmission of refractive errors within Eskimo families. Am J Optom Arch Am Acad Optom 1969;46:676–685.

Zadnik K, Mutti DO. Incidence and Distribution of Refractive Anomalies. In WJ Benjamin (ed), Borish's Clinical Refraction. Philadelphia: Saunders, 1998.

Zylbermann R, Landau D, Berson D. The influence of study habits on myopia in Jewish teenagers. J Pediatr Ophthalmol Strabism 1993;30:319–322.

CHAPTER 3

Clinical Examination

Symptoms of Myopia

In the absence of significant astigmatism or a binocular vision problem, the only symptom of uncorrected myopia is blurred distance vision. If uncorrected myopia is accompanied by astigmatism of 0.50 D or more, symptoms of asthenopia such as headaches and ocular discomfort may also be present. If uncorrected myopia is accompanied by a binocular vision anomaly, the symptoms—headaches, ocular fatigue, diplopia—depend on the specific binocular vision anomaly that is present.

Blurred Distance Vision

When myopia has its onset during the childhood years, a child may not be aware that distance vision is blurred unless he or she is unable to see a distant object that another person can see—such as the writing on a chalkboard—or fails a visual acuity examination. When the onset of myopia occurs during the teen or early adult years, the earliest symptom may be a blurring of distance vision following prolonged near work: This is the *pseudomyopia* stage, which often occurs as a precursor to "real" myopia.

Relationship Between Myopia and Distance Visual Acuity

For a given amount of myopia, unaided distance visual acuity tends to vary widely from one individual to another. Among the factors accounting for this variation are (1) differences in pupil size (the smaller the pupil, the better the acuity for an out-of-focus eye); (2) failure to relax accommodation while fixating a distant object; (3) the tendency for some people to squint, converting the pupil to a narrow slit and thus improving acuity; (4) variations in the aberrations of the eye; and (5) variations in the retinal gradient.

TABLE 3.1
Variation in Unaided Visual Acuity (mean and 95% confidence limits)
for Various Amounts of Myopia

	Unaided Visual Acuity	
Myopia (D)	*Mean*	*95% Confidence Limits*
–0.50	20/25	20/13 to 20/50
–1.00	20/65	20/30 to 20/150
–1.50	20/110	20/50 to 20/250
–2.00	20/165	20/75 to 20/380
–2.50	20/215	20/100 to 20/500
–3.00	20/285	20/130 to 20/650
–4.00	20/420	20/200 to 20/950

Source: Data from MJ Hirsch. Relation of visual acuity to myopia. Arch Ophthalmol
1945;24:418–421.

Hirsch (1945) published data relating myopia and unaided visual acuity, based on an analysis of clinic records of 64 eyes of college students having myopia from –0.50 to –13.50 D. As shown in Table 3.1, visual acuity (95% confidence limits) ranged from 20/13 to 20/60 for myopia of –0.50 D, from 20/30 to 20/150 for myopia of –1.00 D, and from 20/75 to 20/380 for myopia of –2.00 D.

The relationship of unaided visual acuity with both spherical ametropia and astigmatism was investigated at three age levels by Peters (1961). Data were taken from the clinic records of 2,452 eyes of patients ages 5–15 years, from 2,626 eyes of patients ages 25–35 years, and from 2,183 eyes of patients ages 45–55 years. For each age group, Peters published graphs showing visual acuity as a function of spherical refractive error (both myopia and hyperopia) and astigmatism. For the myopic eyes, mean visual acuity for a given amount of myopia and astigmatism did not vary for the three age groups. As shown in Table 3.2, taken from Peters's graphs, mean acuity for various amounts of spherical error differed little from the data published by Hirsch (1945), but each 0.50 D of astigmatism accounted for a decrease in acuity from one to two lines of letters.

Causes of Blurred Distance Vision
Other Than Myopia

Congenital or Developmental Conditions
Very rarely, a child who complains of blurred distance vision is found on ophthalmoscopy to have a previously undiagnosed congenital or developmental anomaly of the retina or optic nerve or functional amblyopia. For this reason, a conclusion that a child who complains of blurred distance vision is myopic is only tentative until a refraction and an ocular health examination have been done.

TABLE 3.2
Mean Unaided Visual Acuity for Various Amounts of Myopia and Astigmatism

Myopia (DS)	Astigmatism (DC)	Unaided Acuity
–0.50	0.00	20/30
	–0.50	20/45
	–1.00	20/60
–1.00	0.00	20/60
	–0.50	20/70
	–1.00	20/80
–1.50	0.00	20/80
	–0.50	20/100
	–1.00	20/150
–2.00	0.00	20/200

DC = diopters cylinder; DS = diopters sphere.
Source: Data from HB Peters. The relationship between refractive error and visual acuity at three age levels. Am J Optom Arch Am Acad Optom 1961;38:194–197.

Lens Changes

When a middle-aged or older patient complains of blurred distance vision, the possibility of myopia secondary to crystalline lens changes should be considered. The two most common causes of lens changes in this age group are nuclear cataracts and incipient diabetes. If only one eye has blurred distance vision, the likely cause is a nuclear cataract, which often occurs first in one eye and then in the other, whereas diabetes would be expected to cause blurred distance vision and myopia in both eyes.

☼ Clinical Pearl

A complaint of blurred distance vision almost always indicates the presence of uncorrected or undercorrected myopia or myopic astigmatism. However, it is possible that blurred distance vision in a child is due to a congenital or developmental anomaly such as functional amblyopia and that blurred distance vision in a middle-aged or older adult may be due to nuclear cataract or diabetes.

Symptoms Due to Binocular Vision Anomalies

Anomalies of binocular vision, which may accompany uncorrected myopia, include heterophorias, strabismus, and anomalies of accommodation.

Heterophorias

When uncorrected myopia is accompanied by a heterophoria, the symptoms (if any) depend on whether the phoria is in the exo or eso direction, and whether it occurs for distance or near fixation, or both.

Exophoria

As with a patient who is emmetropic or hyperopic, symptoms of occasional diplopia at distance in an uncorrected myope usually indicate a distance exophoria. If a significant exophoria is present *only* for distance fixation, the condition is described as *divergence excess.* If an uncorrected myope complains of visual fatigue accompanying prolonged near work, the practitioner may find a nearpoint exophoria; if a significant exophoria occurs *only* during near fixation, the condition is *convergence insufficiency.* Symptoms of eyestrain and occasional diplopia for *both* distance and near tasks should lead the practitioner to expect to find a *basic exophoria*—that is, exophoria at both distance and near.

It is obvious that the symptoms described above would indicate a *habitual* exophoria, as measured in the uncorrected state. Because minus lenses are expected to increase the amount of accommodation and therefore the amount of accommodative convergence, the *induced phoria*, taken through the lenses correcting the refractive error, would be less exo, or even ortho or eso, depending on the amount of myopia and the relationship between accommodative convergence and accommodation (the AC/A ratio).

Esophoria

Previously uncorrected or undercorrected myopes are often found to have a nearpoint esophoria when tested through the subjective lenses. As explained by Flom and Takahashi (1962), this is because in the uncorrected or undercorrected state, a smaller amount of accommodation (and thus accommodative convergence) is required than is required for an emmetrope, resulting in a nearpoint exophoria: This exophoria is compensated by relative convergence (positive fusional vergence), which becomes conditioned, and when the full amount of minus power is prescribed, this conditioned convergence remains and results in a nearpoint esophoria. After a short time, however, this nearpoint esophoria decreases in amount or even disappears. For 14 previously uncorrected or undercorrected myopes who had a nearpoint esophoria at the initial examination, Flom and Takahashi found that after a week or longer the nearpoint esophoria reduced by an average of 3Δ, and the distance esophoria reduced by an average of less than 1Δ. Because the patient was *orthophoric* or *exophoric* in the uncorrected or undercorrected state, symptoms such as headaches or eyestrain are not expected in the initial case history, but they might be reported once the full minus lenses are worn.

If, for a newly corrected myope who is found to have a nearpoint esophoria, the esophoria fails to materially decrease or disappear within about a week, it may cause symptoms of headaches or eyestrain.

Vertical Phoria

A common symptom of a vertical phoria is a vertical diplopia. Whenever a patient has a complaint of double vision, the patient should be asked whether the two objects are separated vertically or horizontally, and also whether the double vision occurs for distance vision or for near vision or both. Another common symptom of vertical phoria is skipping lines when reading.

Strabismus

Because of adaptations including suppression, amblyopia, and anomalous retinal correspondence, a long-standing strabismus—whether it accompanies myopia, emmetropia, or hyperopia—is seldom a source of patient symptoms. An exception to this general rule may occur when a strabismus accompanied by diplopia manifests itself only for distance fixation or for near fixation. A newly acquired strabismus, particularly in an adult, may be the source of an intractable diplopia.

Anomalies of Accommodation

Anomalies of accommodation that may occur in conjunction with myopia include spasm of accommodation, infacility of accommodation, fatigue of accommodation, accommodative insufficiency, and, of course, presbyopia.

Spasm of Accommodation (Pseudomyopia)
As noted earlier, the earliest symptom of myopia may be a blurring of distance vision following prolonged near work due to failure to relax accommodation. This distance blur may clear up after a few minutes, or it may persist.

Infacility of Accommodation
The inability to quickly increase or decrease the amount of accommodation in play can occur in myopia, but it is not likely to be a source of symptoms that would be reported by a myopic patient during the history.

Fatigue of Accommodation
A complaint of eyestrain or fatigue accompanying near work may result from a deficient accommodative response, which is often found in incipient myopia. However, in *uncorrected* myopia the need for accommodation is reduced, so a deficient accommodative response is not likely to be a source of symptoms. A deficient accommodative response can be confirmed by tests of the lag of accommodation such as dynamic retinoscopy and the binocular crossed-cylinder test.

Accommodative Insufficiency
A reduced amplitude of accommodation may be present in a myopic child or young adult, but it is not likely to be a source of symptoms. Because an uncorrected myope has less need to accommodate than an emmetrope, on initial testing there may be a lowered amplitude, but the amplitude will usually increase with the wearing of minus lenses. Another sign of accom-

modative insufficiency is a high lag of accommodation. As discussed in Chapter 4, a potential treatment for high lag cases is a plus add for near.

Paralysis of Accommodation
This is a rare condition, which has no predilection for myopia. Of the 10 causes of paralysis of accommodation described by Duke-Elder (1947), he noted that the most common cause is accidental instillation of *a cyclo-plegic drug.*

Presbyopia
With the exception of myopia secondary to nuclear cataracts or diabetes, very few people become myopic during the presbyopic years. However, occasionally a person reaches the presbyopic years with a small amount of uncorrected myopia, resulting in the symptoms of presbyopia possibly being delayed for a few years.

☀ **Clinical Pearl**
It should be remembered that a patient may not have just one problem but rather multiple problems. When a patient complains of blurred distance vision—which obviously leads to a tentative diagnosis of myopia—the practitioner should question the patient further concerning symptoms such as headaches, eyestrain, and diplopia, which may indicate the presence of a binocular vision problem.

Refractive Examination

The refractive examination procedure for the myope (or suspected myope on the basis of lowered distance visual acuity) differs little from the routine objective and subjective examination. The one difference is that the examiner must be aware of the possibility of pseudomyopia, just as he or she would be aware of the possibility of latent hyperopia for a patient who has 20/20 or 20/15 entering acuity.

Keratometry

Even though any existing astigmatism will be found in retinoscopy or subjective refraction, it is worth taking the 2 or 3 minutes necessary to perform keratometry, for several reasons: (1) due to small pupils, squinting or poor patient responses, small (or even moderate) amounts of astigmatism may be missed in retinoscopy or subjective testing; (2) keratoconus and other corneal anomalies can be easily ruled out; (3) the estimated total astigmatism can be easily determined by combining the cylinder lens required to correct the keratometric astigmatism with –0.50 x 090. For example, for the keratometer finding

42.00 @ 180; 43.25 @ 090,

the lens required to correct the keratometric astigmatism is

$$-1.25 \text{ DC} \times 180,$$

and the estimated total astigmatism is therefore

$$-0.75 \text{ DC} \times 180.$$

Retinoscopy

In performing static retinoscopy, it is important to make sure that the patient is actually fixating the letter on the acuity chart or other distant object that is presented. Some patients, particularly children, have a strong tendency to look at the retinoscope light source, because it is the brightest object in the room. It is a good idea for the examiner not only to instruct the patient to "tell me if my head gets in the way of the chart," but also to test the patient's responses by occasionally moving his or her head so that it *is in the way of the chart.*

Experience has shown that when static retinoscopy is performed on large numbers of children in a vision screening test, many children who have read 20/20 or better on the Snellen chart will be found by retinoscopy to have as much as 0.50 or 1.00 D of "myopia," due to the accommodation not being fully relaxed.

Subjective Refraction

If myopia is suspected on the basis of symptoms, unaided acuity, or retinoscopy, subjective refraction need not differ from the usual procedure with the exception that the examiner should make sure that the binocular subjective endpoint is approached by "coming out of the fog," using the criterion "maximum plus or minimum minus for best visual acuity." In comparing the results of retinoscopy and subjective refraction, it should be recalled that because retinoscopy is a *monocular* test, in which only the eye not being examined is presented with a distant object to fixate, there is less control of accommodation than there is during the determination of the binocular subjective endpoint.

Pseudomyopia

The typical pseudomyope, despite complaints of blurred distance vision after prolonged near work, has unaided visual acuity of 20/20 or better and typically will accept a small amount of minus sphere on retinoscopy but will accept less minus sphere or plano (or even a small amount of plus power) on the binocular subjective endpoint.

It is important to recognize pseudomyopia when it is present, because at this stage the patient's myopia may be more amenable to control procedures (discussed in the following chapters), including visual hygiene, vision therapy, and the use of a plus add for near work.

Binocular Vision Examination

As with any patient, binocular vision tests for a myopic or suspected myopic patient should be performed with care. It is false economy to save a few minutes of examination time by failing to perform one or more of the important tests for binocular vision. Undoubtedly, the most important binocular vision test is the *cover test* or *cover tests*, if we consider the unilateral and alternating cover tests to be separate tests. Other tests of importance are the von Graefe dissociated phoria test, tests of fusional vergence reserves, and associated phoria tests.

Cover Tests

Compared with the von Graefe phoria test, which is commonly done while the patient is behind the refractor, the cover test has the advantage that it is done in open space, which of course is necessary to be able to observe the patients' eyes. The absence of lens apertures has the additional advantage that there is no stimulus to proximal accommodation and convergence.

It has been shown by Rainey et al. (1998a) that for experienced practitioners, estimating the phoria by means of the alternating cover test will provide results that are very close to the results obtained with von Graefe phoria testing. However, results by Calvin et al. (1996) have shown that for final year optometry students, estimated cover test results (although correlating well with von Graefe phoria results) occasionally underestimate the von Graefe phoria by clinically significant amounts.

Unilateral Cover Test

The unilateral cover test is performed to rule out a tropia (strabismus). While the patient wears his or her habitual correction (if any), the examiner instructs the patient to fixate a single letter on the Snellen chart at 6 m (or on a handheld reduced Snellen chart at 40 cm), and covers one eye for a period of approximately 1 second. When the cover is placed on the eye, the examiner intently watches the eye that is not covered and continues to watch the not-covered eye while the cover is removed. Any movement of the not-covered eye indicates a tropia: If the not-covered eye moves outward to take up fixation when the fellow eye is covered, this indicates an esotropia, whereas an inward movement indicates exotropia. The cover is then placed on the opposite eye, and the procedure is repeated. The entire procedure is then repeated, at least once. If a tropia is found at either 6 m or 40 cm, it is recorded in terms of the deviating eye, for example, right esotropia, left exotropia. With experience, the examiner will learn to estimate the amount of the tropia and may record the finding as, for example, 4Δ *exotropia*. However, the student clinician or recent graduate is advised to record the results simply as, for example, *exotropia*, or *low exotropia*.

Alternating Cover Test

The alternating cover test detects either a tropia or a phoria, but does not distinguish between the two; however, if a tropia has not been found on the unilateral cover test, any movement seen on the alternating cover test indicates the presence of a phoria. As with the unilateral cover test, the patient wears his or her habitual correction (if any), and the examiner instructs the patient to fixate a single letter on the Snellen chart at 6 m (or on a handheld reduced Snellen chart at 40 cm). One eye is covered for a period of approximately 1 second, and the occluder is then quickly moved to the other eye, where it remains for approximately 1 second. The entire test is then repeated. As the examiner moves the occluder from one eye to the other, he or she intently watches the just-uncovered eye: If the eye moves outward when the cover is removed and placed on the fellow eye, the condition is esophoria (or esotropia); an inward movement indicates exophoria (or exotropia).

Subjective Cover Test

To ensure the patient's cooperation, the examiner should ask the patient two questions: (1) Does the letter on the chart move when I move the paddle from one eye to the other? (2) Which way does it move, in the same direction as the movement of my paddle or in the opposite direction? With children (and even with adults), the patient's decision is simplified if he or she is asked to move both thumbs back and forth, in the direction of the movement of the letter. The examiner then simply watches the thumbs to determine if the movement is in the same or opposite direction as that of the cover paddle. The subjective cover test result could be recorded as a separate test, but normally the patient's response is taken into consideration, along with the examiner's observation, and a single cover test recording is made.

If the patient is found to have strabismus on the unilateral cover test, the subjective alternating cover test should not be performed, because a strabismic patient who has harmonious anomalous retinal correspondence will not observe any movement of the fixated object on the alternating cover test.

Prism-Neutralized Cover Test

If a tropia or a phoria has been found on the unilateral or alternating cover test, the deviation can easily be measured by the use of a prism-bar or handheld prisms. The alternating cover test is repeated while a measuring prism is held in front of one eye. A recommended method is to initially increase the amount of prism power in 4Δ increments; each time a prism is interposed, the examiner intently watches the just-uncovered eye and notes whether eso or exo movement occurs. For example, if on the original cover test the examiner noted that the just-uncovered eye moved outward by an estimated 6Δ (indicating approximately 6Δ of esophoria), he or she would first place a 4Δ prism, base-out, in front of one eye, and repeat the test. If outward (eso) movement was still observed, the test would be repeated with an 8Δ prism, base-out; if this resulted in inward (exo) movement, the test would be repeated with a 6Δ prism, base-out; and if no movement was observed, the test result would be recorded as 6Δ *esophoria*.

The argument can be made that the result of the prism-neutralized cover test should be more accurate than that of the von Graefe phoria test, for reasons already mentioned: The examiner can observe the patient's eyes, and there are no lens apertures to stimulate proximal accommodation or convergence.

von Graefe Dissociated Phoria Test

The von Graefe test is routinely performed, at 6 m and at 40 cm, with the best visual acuity (BVA) lenses in the refractor. A dissociating prism of 7 or 8Δ, base-down, is placed in front of one eye, and it is crucial that the patient keep the line of letters on the distance or near chart in sharp focus as the measuring Risley prism is slowly (but not too slowly) reduced from a starting point of approximately 15Δ base-in. The patient is asked to report when one line of letters is directly above the other line.

"Flash" Method

Using the "flash" method, the patient is initially asked to report whether the upper line of letters is *to the right*, *to the left*, or *right above* the lower line. If the dissociating prism is placed base-up in front of the left eye, the letters seen with that eye appear to be above those seen with the right eye (unless a large vertical phoria exists). With the 15Δ base-in measuring prism in front of the right eye, the patient (unless highly exophoric) reports that the upper line of letters is *to the right* of the lower line. The right eye is occluded and the measuring prism is reduced to, say 10Δ, the occluder is quickly removed, and the question is asked again. If additional reductions of approximately 5–7Δ are made, only two or three changes have to be made until the patient reports *to the left*, following which the prism power is reduced, in smaller steps, until the patient reports *right above*.

Many practitioners prefer the flash method to the classic von Graefe method, because the patient is less likely to make positive or negative fusional vergence movements when he or she is permitted to see both lines of letters for only a brief moment.

Other Measures of Dissociated Phoria

Other methods of measuring dissociated phorias include the Maddox rod and the modified Thorington test (Daum, 1991; Schroeder et al., 1996). The modified Thorington test, despite being uncommonly used, appears to be the most reliable method of dissociated phoria measurement (Rainey et al., 1998b).

Tests of Fusional Vergence Reserves

If a significant phoria (more than 2Δ or 3Δ) is found with the prism-neutralized cover test or the von Graefe dissociated phoria test, tests of positive and negative fusional vergence reserves should be performed. These tests are valuable because they provide an indication of how well the visual system is compensating for the phoria.

Negative Fusional Vergence Reserve

With the BVA subjective lenses in place, the patient is presented with a vertical line of 20/20 letters on the 6-m or 40-cm chart and is asked to report when the letters *begin to blur* and then when they *break into two lines of letters,* as the power of the Risley prisms (starting with zero base-in) is gradually increased in the base-in direction. The total amount of prism power (for both prisms) is recorded if the patient reports a blur (which is not expected on this test at 6 m), and then reports a break. The patient is then asked to report when the *two lines come back together,* as the base-in prism is slowly reduced, and the total amount of prism in place at that point is recorded as the recovery.

Positive Fusional Vergence Reserve

This test is done in the same manner as the negative fusional vergence reserve test, with the exception that the Risley prisms are moved in the base-out direction, rather than base-in. Because a test requiring convergence may cause some "spill-over" into a test requiring divergence due to prism adaptation, the base-in test is routinely performed *before* the base-out test (Rosenfield et al., 1995; Goss, 1995).

Associated Phoria Tests

Tests of associated phorias, sometimes incorrectly referred to as *fixation disparity tests,* are designed to determine the oculomotor balance when both eyes are presented with the same object of fixation (i.e., the eyes are not dissociated). The main advantage of these tests, according to their proponents, is that the amount of prism that measures the associated phoria (i.e., the amount of prism that eliminates the fixation disparity) is the amount of prism to be prescribed. Some of the proponents of these tests recommend that when such a test is done, dissociated phoria and fusional vergence reserve tests need not be done.

Fixation Disparity Tests

Also currently available are tests that are designed to measure fixation disparity, rather than determine the prism power necessary to eliminate the fixation disparity. Such tests include the Sheedy Disparometer and the Wesson Fixation Disparity Card.

Analysis and prescribing on the basis of the results of dissociated phoria tests, fusional vergence reserve tests, associated phoria tests, and fixation disparity tests are presented in Chapter 4.

 Clinical Pearl

Due to the fact that optometrists currently have the responsibility of using diagnostic and therapeutic drugs in all 50 states in the United States, there is sometimes a temptation to do a "quick refraction" and then move on to the dilation. However, the demographics are such that if optometrists fail to maintain expertise in the areas of optics, refraction, and binocular vision, most will end up with very little to do!

Ocular Health Examination

Because myopic eyes are at a greater risk than emmetropic or hyperopic eyes for a number of disease conditions such as vitreous detachment, retinal detachment, chorioretinal degeneration, and open-angle glaucoma, they should be given a comprehensive ocular health examination including direct ophthalmoscopy, biomicroscopy, tonometry, visual field screening, and dilated fundus examination using binocular indirect ophthalmoscopy. When the patient is a child, it is often preferable to schedule the more time-consuming procedures such as visual field screening and the dilated fundus examination for a return visit.

Direct Ophthalmoscopy

Due to the current emphasis on dilated fundus examination—which is impractical to perform until after the completion of tests of refraction and binocular vision—many currently practicing optometrists have been taught *not* to use the direct ophthalmoscope as a part of the preliminary examination. A problem with this method is that if an eye should have a congenital fundus abnormality, a degenerative lesion, or a cataract, its presence will not be known at the time the refractive and binocular vision examinations are done. It is recommended, therefore, that undilated direct ophthalmoscopy should be performed as a part of the preliminary examination.

Because of the high magnification afforded by the direct ophthalmoscope, changes in the central (posterior) fundus may sometimes be detected more readily with this instrument than with the binocular indirect ophthalmoscope. However, the many sight-threatening changes that may occur in the peripheral fundus of a myopic eye require the extended field of view, the increased brightness, and the stereoscopic vision that are available with the binocular indirect ophthalmoscope.

The pathologic changes that may occur in posterior fundus of a myopic eye and thus can be detected with the direct ophthalmoscope—optic nerve crescents, localized tessellation and pallor indicating a posterior staphyloma, small retinal hemorrhages, lacquer cracks, focal areas of atrophy, peripapillary atrophy, subretinal neovascular membranes, and Fuchs' spot—are described in Chapter 1.

Biomicroscopy

Routine biomicroscopy, an important part of the ocular health examination, is neither more nor less important for myopic eyes than for emmetropic or hyperopic eyes. Expected biomicroscopic findings in the myopic eye are a relatively deep anterior chamber with a wide-open angle. Using the Van Herick angle-grading system, the eyes of young myopes typically have grade 4 angles, which may gradually reduce to grade 3 during the adult years. An advantage of the wide-open angle typically found in a myopic eye is that there is very seldom a risk of angle-closure when dilating drops are instilled. An exception to this general rule may be a reduction in angle width due to swelling of the lens in an incipient cataract.

Tonometry

As with emmetropic and hyperopic eyes, applanation tonometry should not be neglected when examining a myope. Although there may be some reluctance to perform tonometry on a child, experience shows that for most children the expert use of a Goldmann or handheld applanation tonometer is more successful than the use of an "air-puff" tonometer.

Visual Field Screening

Some form of visual field screening should be a part of every comprehensive examination. Because the majority of lesions causing visual field losses affect the central field before they affect the peripheral field, the screening procedure should involve a method of central field testing such as the use of a tangent screen or one of the programmed visual field screeners.

Dilated Fundus Examination

Many of the conditions that may be found as a result of a dilated fundus examination are much more likely to occur in a myopic eye than in an emmetropic or hyperopic eye. As described in Chapter 1, these include vitreoretinal traction, cystoid degeneration, lattice degeneration, paving stone degeneration, pigmentary degeneration, and retinal holes and tears. The management of patients who have fundus anomalies and other complications of myopia is discussed in Chapter 5.

☼ Clinical Pearl

Optometrists have traditionally taken the responsibility of providing primary vision care for the great majority of myopic patients. With the ever-expanding role of optometric practice during the past decades, optometrists are obliged not only to maintain their expertise in the traditional optometric care of myopes but also to develop and maintain expertise in the diagnosis and management—to the extent possible—of the complications of myopia.

References

Calvin H, Rupnow F, Grosvenor T. How well does the estimated cover test predict the von Graefe phoria measurement? Optom Vis Sci 1996;73:701–706.

Curtin BJ. The Myopias, Basic Science and Clinical Management. Philadelphia: Harper & Row, 1985.

Daum KM. Heterophoria and Heterotropia. In JB Eskridge, JF Amos, JD Bartlett (eds), Clinical Procedures in Optometry. Philadelphia: Lippincott, 1991.

Duke-Elder S. Textbook of Ophthalmology, Vol. IV. St. Louis: Mosby, 1947.

Flom MC, Takahashi E. The AC/A ratio and undercorrected myopia. Am J Optom Arch Am Acad Optom 1962;39:305–312.

Goss DA. Effect of test sequence on fusional vergence ranges. Engl J Optom 1995; 47:39–42.

Hirsch MJ. Relation of visual acuity to myopia. Arch Ophthalmol 1945;24:418–421.

Peters HB. The relationship between refractive error and visual acuity at three age levels. Am J Optom Arch Am Acad Optom 1961;38:194–197.

Rainey BB, Schroeder TL, Goss DA, Grosvenor T. Reliability of three variations of the alternating cover test. Ophthal Physiol Opt 1998a. In press.

Rainey BB, Schroeder TL, Goss DA, Grosvenor T. Inter-examiner reliability of heterophoria tests. Optom Vis Sci 1998b. In press.

Rosenfield M, Ciuffreda KJ, Ong E, Super S. Vergence adaptation and the order of clinical vergence range testing. Optom Vis Sci 1995;72:219–223.

Schroeder TL, Rainey BB, Goss DA, Grosvenor T. A review of studies investigating reliability of and comparisons between methods of measuring dissociated phoria. Optom Vis Sci 1996;73:389–397.

CHAPTER 4

Prescribing for Myopia

In the preface to this book, we made the distinction between myopia correction, myopia control, and myopia reduction. This chapter covers myopia correction—the provision of optical compensation for the myopia to restore normal distance visual acuity. In addition to the restoration of normal distance visual acuity, prescriptions for myopia should also yield comfortable efficient binocular vision. Among the factors to consider in deciding whether to prescribe for myopia and deciding on the power to prescribe are the patient's age, amount of myopia, visual needs, and the presence of other ocular and visual conditions, such as astigmatism, anisometropia, and accommodation and vergence disorders. Patients' visual needs depend on their occupational, educational, and recreational activities. Because each patient presents a unique combination of needs, problems, and test findings, prescribing for myopia requires the clinician's professional judgment. Some basic guidelines, however, can be suggested.

General Guidelines

One of the first considerations is the patient's age. The visual world of infants and toddlers is relatively close to them, so in general myopia of up to approximately 3 D need not be corrected. Another consideration in such cases is that myopic refractive errors of up to 3 D in infancy can potentially reduce to emmetropia by about age 2 years (Gwiazda et al., 1993). Preschool children start to interact with persons and things at intermediate distance, and correction of myopia as low as 1–2 D can be indicated. If the clinician decides not to correct the myopia, regular follow-up at intervals of approximately 6 months are advisable. At these progress checks, the myopia should be corrected if it has increased in amount or if there are signs that poor far or intermediate distance vision has adversely affected the child behaviorally. Once children enter school, distance vision becomes more important because they must be able to read the chalkboard. Thus, clinicians may choose to correct 1.00 D of myopia in first- or second-grade students. It is not necessary to routinely correct low myopia of approximately 0.50 D in grade school children. If children with very low myopia complain of difficulty reading the chalkboard, the clinician may recommend that the teacher move the child to the front of the classroom. Because it is likely that myopia will increase in such cases, these children should be examined again in 6 months.

As children progress through school, demands on distance vision increase; therefore, the minimum amount of myopia that should routinely be corrected decreases. In the adolescent or adult patient, the majority of clinicians will correct any amount of myopia that will improve distance visual acuity. In adults, myopia as low as –0.25 D may be corrected in some cases. The case history is very important in deciding whether to prescribe such low lens power. Patients who are more precise and discriminating may have visual complaints relieved by very low-power prescriptions (Blume, 1987; Brookman, 1996). Patients may also benefit from correction of low amounts of myopia if their occupational, educational, or recreational activities require optimal distance vision (Goss et al., 1998).

As discussed in Chapter 1, increases in myopia are expected in childhood and often occur in adulthood as well. A review of papers on the repeatability of refraction suggests that the 95% limits of agreement for refraction is ±0.50 D (Goss and Grosvenor, 1996); therefore, when refractive error differs from the habitual correction by 0.50 D or more, a change in prescription may be warranted. For patients who are very precise and discriminating, changes as small as 0.25 D may be indicated. Demonstrating to the patient the difference in vision with and without the additional 0.25 D can be helpful in confirming whether new spectacles will be beneficial.

☀ CLINICAL PEARL
The 95% limits of agreement for repeatability of refraction is approximately ±0.50 D, but patients who are very precise about their vision may prefer corrections or changes in corrections of as little as 0.25 D. "Trial framing" is a useful procedure in such cases to confirm the advisability of a low correction or change.

Case Report

A 31-year-old copyeditor complained of a slight blur at distance with her glasses. She had no other eye or vision complaints. She participated in walking and various service organizations in her spare time. Her spectacle correction was –3.25 – 0.50 x 180 OD, –3.50 – 0.25 x 170 OS. Distance visual acuities with that correction were 20/20–²⁄₆ OD and 20/20–¹⁄₆ OS. Subjective refraction was –3.50 – 0.75 x 5 OD and –3.75 – 0.50 x 170 OS. Distance visual acuities with the subjective refraction were 20/15 OD and OS. Phorias with the subjective refraction lenses were 1Δ exo at distance and 3Δ exo at 40 cm. Fusional vergence ranges and relative accommodation findings were all within normal limits. Ocular health was normal.

The refraction indicates a small increase in myopia and a small increase in astigmatism for a spherical equivalent change of –0.37 D in each eye. The patient noticed an improvement in distance vision clarity with the updated prescription, and lenses equal in power to the subjective refraction were ordered. A change of –0.37 D is not a large change, but a fairly precise individual, such as this patient, often will report a definite improvement with that amount of change, and will wish to obtain new lenses to maximize distance vision clarity. Her occupation demands heavy reading and near work. Test findings suggest that she should not have asthenopia at near with the new lenses. She was advised to return for another eye and vision examination in 2 years or earlier if she noticed any vision problems.

Many patients whose myopia may have been inadvertently overcorrected in their habitual correction adapt to the overcorrection, and claim they can see more clearly with the overcorrection than with an exact correction. Some clinicians recommend reducing the minus correction in such cases, and carefully educating the patient about the need to reduce the minus prescription. Other clinicians do not reduce the minus because of the successful adaptation, waiting until the patient experiences symptoms of accommodative problems to make the change to a lower minus power. If either the theory that optical defocus induces myopia or the theory that the process of accommodation causes myopia is correct, reducing any overcorrection of myopia may aid in slowing future increases in myopia.

For patients with compound myopic astigmatism, cylindrical correction should generally be included with the lens prescription whenever the astigmatic error is 0.50 D or more. Patients with 0.25 D of astigmatism generally do not need a 0.25 D cylinder included in their prescription, except when a prior comfortable prescription incorporated a 0.25 D cylinder. As a general rule, low amounts of uncorrected against-the-rule astigmatism are more likely to be associated with ocular symptoms than are low amounts of with-the-rule astigmatism.

Accommodation and Vergence Considerations

As noted, the clinician should be concerned with more than just the restoration of clear distance vision. Comfortable, efficient binocular vision must also be a primary consideration. In many cases, lenses that restore clear distance vision are not the most appropriate lenses for efficient near vision. A careful evaluation of accommodation and vergence function is an important part of management of the patient with myopia. As a general rule, guidelines for management of accommodation and vergence disorders are readily applied for patients with myopia (Cooper, 1987; Wick, 1987; Birnbaum, 1993; Scheiman and Wick, 1994; Goss, 1995, 1996a,b). Nearpoint plus lens additions are often appropriate for patients with convergence excess or accommodative insufficiency.

Convergence Excess

Test findings typical of convergence excess include normal distance phoria, esophoria at near, high accommodative convergence–to–accommodation (AC/A) ratio, low base-in fusional vergence range at near, and low positive relative accommodation (PRA). Convergence excess patients also often have a higher than normal lag of accommodation, because a decrease in accommodation is associated with the divergence necessary for single vision in esophoria. A common method for deriving the lens add power in convergence excess is to find the add that shifts the near phoria to ortho or low exo. For example, consider the patient with orthophoria at distance, 7Δ esophoria at 40 cm through the subjective refraction, and 1Δ esophoria at 40 cm through a +1.00 D add. The calculated AC/A ratio would be $8.8\Delta/D$, determined as follows:

$$\text{Calculated AC/A} = \frac{\dfrac{\text{Convergence stimulus}}{\text{of near target}} - \dfrac{\text{distance}}{\text{phoria}} + \dfrac{\text{near}}{\text{phoria}}}{\text{Accommodative stimulus of near target}}$$

where esophoria is plus and exophoria is minus

$$\text{Calculated AC/A} = \frac{15\Delta - 0\Delta + 7\Delta}{2.50 \text{ D}} = 8.8\Delta/D$$

The gradient AC/A ratio is $6\Delta/D$:

$$\text{Gradient AC/A ratio} = \begin{pmatrix}\text{Phoria at near with} \\ \text{subjective refraction}\end{pmatrix} - \begin{pmatrix}\text{Phoria at near with} \\ \text{+1.00 D add}\end{pmatrix}$$

Gradient AC/A ratio = $7 - 1 = 6\Delta/D$

Using the gradient AC/A ratio, the plus add that would achieve orthophoria would be about as follows:

$$\text{Add for ortho} = \frac{\text{Esophoria at near through subjective refraction}}{\text{Gradient AC/A ratio}}$$

$$\text{Add for ortho} = \frac{7\Delta}{6\Delta/D} = 1.17 \text{ D}$$

A plus add for near of +1.25 D therefore should shift the near phoria into the normal range of ortho and low exo. If the patient does not give reliable responses on phoria testing, another method for estimating the proper add is to find the minimum plus add that reduces a near eso fixation disparity to zero. Devices that can be used for this include the Wesson Fixation Disparity Card, the Mallett unit, the Sheedy Disparometer, and the Bernell

Test Lantern near binocular refraction slide (Goss, 1991; Saladin, 1998). Another method for deriving add power is to determine the plus add that balances the negative relative accommodation (NRA) and the PRA (Birnbaum, 1993), although this may not necessarily eliminate the esophoria.

Accommodative Insufficiency

Accommodative insufficiency is characterized by a high lag of accommodation or a low amplitude of accommodation. Other findings in accommodative insufficiency can include a low PRA finding and a slow response on the minus side on lens rock accommodative facility testing. The power of the near plus lens add in accommodative insufficiency and often in convergence excess can be determined by subtracting 0.25 D from the lag of accommodation measured with monocular estimate method (MEM) dynamic retinoscopy or Nott dynamic retinoscopy, or by finding the plus add that balances the NRA and PRA test results. With MEM retinoscopy, the lag of accommodation is estimated by judging the speed, width, and brightness of the retinoscopic reflex (Rouse et al., 1982; Haynes, 1985; Daum, 1991; Saladin, 1998). The patient views a nearpoint target while the examiner performs retinoscopy, usually by viewing through a hole in a specially designed test card. The fixation target and the retinoscope are maintained in the same plane. A plus lens equal in power to the estimated lag can be quickly interposed in front of the patient to confirm the estimate of the lag.

In Nott retinoscopy, the patient again views a nearpoint card, but the retinoscope is moved independently of the test card. The examiner observes whether there is a lag or lead of accommodation present. If a lag of accommodation is observed, the examiner moves the retinoscope back until neutral is observed. The distance of the retinoscope from the spectacle plane is then converted into the accommodative response. The lag of accommodation is the difference between the accommodative stimulus and the accommodative response. For example, a patient views a test card 40 cm from the spectacle plane, and the examiner moves back to 50 cm from the spectacle plane for neutrality. The accommodative stimulus is 1/0.4 m, or 2.50 D. The accommodative response is 1/0.5 m, or 2.00 D. The lag of accommodation in this example is 2.50 D − 2.00 D = 0.50 D. Most nonpresbyopic patients have lags of accommodation as measured by MEM or Nott dynamic retinoscopy in the range of 0 to +0.75 D.

Some clinicians emphasize basing the near add on the lens power, which maximizes the results on performance tests done outside of instruments, for example, performance tests such as near visual acuity, near ranges of clear vision, cover test, nearpoint of convergence, pursuit and saccadic eye movements, stereopsis, and dynamic retinoscopy (Apell, 1996). Another treatment option for accommodative insufficiency is vision therapy. The success rate of vision therapy for accommodative insufficiency is high (Daum, 1983a,b; Suchoff and Petito, 1986; Rouse, 1987).

Pseudoconvergence Insufficiency

Pseudoconvergence insufficiency, or false convergence insufficiency, is a case in which exophoria at near is secondary to accommodative insufficiency (Richman and Cron, 1987; Scheiman and Wick, 1994; Goss, 1995, 1996a). The patient appears to have exophoria at near because the patient does not accommodate adequately, and, therefore, less accommodative convergence is occurring. Like a "true" convergence insufficiency, there is high exophoria at near and a receded nearpoint of convergence. Unlike a true convergence insufficiency, there is a high lag of accommodation and the nearpoint of convergence often improves with a plus add. Unlike a true convergence insufficiency, the base-out fusional vergence range is sometimes normal. Even though it seems paradoxical to prescribe a plus add for a patient with exophoria at near, a plus add is indicated in pseudoconvergence insufficiency, because the exophoria is secondary to the accommodative insufficiency. The power of the plus add can be determined as discussed above for accommodative insufficiency.

Many patients and parents are unaware that bifocals or progressive addition lenses can be indicated for nonpresbyopes. Patient acceptance of such lenses is improved if enhanced clarity of near vision or better nearpoint performance is demonstrated before discussing multifocal lenses. If the patient or parents are aware that the patient will benefit from different lens powers for distance and near, the reason for the multifocal lenses becomes clear. If the recommended add power is close to the amount of the patient's myopia and the patient has minimal amounts of astigmatism and anisometropia, another option for a nearpoint plus add is removing the minus lens spectacles when reading and doing near work.

☼ CLINICAL PEARL

A nearpoint plus add usually improves near work efficiency of patients with convergence excess or accommodative insufficiency. Such nearpoint plus adds can be provided in bifocals or progressive addition lenses, or in cases of low myopia, minimal astigmatism, and minimal anisometropia by removing the distance correction glasses.

Case Report

A 12-year-old noticed that he could not read the chalkboard at school as well as his friends could. He did not report blur or discomfort during near work. He had not had a previous eye and vision examination. He excelled in school. He enjoyed reading, and often read for pleasure outside of school. His hobbies included collecting stamps with his father and playing soccer and basketball. His unaided visual acuities were 20/80 OD and OS at distance, and 20/20 OD and OS at near. Cover test with no correction showed ortho at distance and a very slight exophoria at near. The subjective refraction revealed –1.25 D sphere OD and –1.25 D sphere OS. These lenses yielded distance visual acuities of 20/20 OD and OS. Phorias with correction using the von Graefe method were ortho at distance and 3Δ eso at 40 cm. The +1.00 D gradient phoria was 3Δ exo. Fusional vergence ranges were X/7/3 base-in and 12/20/10 base-out at distance, and 10/19/11 base-in and X/22/14 base-out at 40 cm. NRA was +2.25 D and PRA was –1.00 D. Ocular health was normal in each eye.

Minus lenses were prescribed to improve the patient's distance visual acuity. Because of his esophoria at near, he was advised to remove his glasses when he read for long periods. This would effectively be a +1.25 D add and would shift the near phoria into a small amount of exo. Based on the +1.00 D gradient phoria, lower adds would make the near phoria normal, but removing glasses for reading for long periods was considered a viable option to the use of a multifocal lens. The low PRA was also an indication for a plus add at near. The nature of childhood myopia progression was explained to the parents, and it was recommended that another examination be performed in a year. This is a very typical case of the initial examination of a child who has developed myopia.

Basic Exophoria

Basic exophoria is characterized by high exophoria of about the same amount at distance and near. Because the phorias are about the same at distance and near, the AC/A ratio is in the moderate range. Base-out fusional vergence ranges are usually low at distance and near. The PRA may be low. If a patient with basic exophoria has normal accommodative function, full-time use of the full correction of the myopia may be advisable. The rationale for this recommendation is that without spectacle correction the patient would have an even higher exophoria at near.

Divergence Excess

Divergence excess is characterized by high exophoria at distance and a normal phoria at near. The patient thus has a high AC/A ratio. There is a considerable range of opinions on the nature, diagnosis, and treatment of divergence excess (Wick, 1987; Scheiman and Wick, 1994; Griffin and Grisham, 1995; Cooper, 1996; Flax, 1996; Rutstein and Daum, 1998; Newman, 1998). Some have suggested that there are subtypes of divergence excess. If we consider only the most general case in which there is high exo at distance, a normal amount of exophoria at near, and a high AC/A ratio, it is usually appropriate to prescribe a full correction for myopia. In young patients whose high distance exo deviation is an intermittent exotropia, an overcorrection for myopia may be provided to promote fusion through the use of accommodative convergence until vision therapy to improve positive fusional vergence and sensory fusion has been undertaken.

Convergence Insufficiency

In the classic presentation of convergence insufficiency, the distance phoria is normal and the near phoria is high exo. The AC/A ratio is low. Accommodation is normal. The nearpoint of convergence is receded, and the base-out fusional vergence range at near is low. Some clinicians rely most on the endpoint and the patient's ease of performance on the nearpoint of convergence test to make a diagnosis of convergence insufficiency. Because the AC/A ratio is so low in convergence insufficiency, altering the lens prescription does not have a great effect on the phoria status. The treatment of choice for convergence insufficiency is vision therapy, which has a very high rate of success (Cooper and Duckman, 1978; Cooper et al., 1983; Suchoff and Petito, 1986; Daum, 1986; Griffin, 1987; Grisham, 1988). Signs, symptoms, and management of common binocular vision problems are summarized in Table 4.1.

Presbyopia

The guidelines for management of presbyopia (Patorgis, 1987; Kurtz, 1996) for patients with myopia are essentially the same as those for patients with emmetropia, with two exceptions. One minor exception is that the accommodative stimulus for a spectacle-corrected myope is somewhat less than that for an emmetrope and for a spectacle-corrected hyperope. For example, the principal plane stimulus to accommodation for a fixation object 40 cm from the spectacle plane is 2.18 D for a 3.00 D myope with the correcting lens at a vertex distance of 14 mm and an assumed distance of 1.35 mm from the corneal apex to the principal plane, compared with 2.41 D for an emmetrope and 2.64 D for a 3.00 D hyperope. The difference increases as the amount of ametropia increases. The difference also increases as the vertex distance increases. A consequence of this is that patients with significant amounts of anisometropia may require a slightly higher add in the more myopic eye. Before prescribing unequal adds, however, appropriate testing and trial frame confirmation should be performed. Because of lens effectiveness of minus lenses, patients with moderate to high amounts of myopia can have a slight improvement in near vision clarity by increasing the vertex distance of the spectacles.

Another difference between presbyopia for myopes and presbyopia for emmetropes and hyperopes is that the patient with myopia can remove his or her distance glasses for reading. Some patients prefer this situation, although others find bifocals or progressive addition lenses more convenient than having to remove their glasses for reading. The option of removing the glasses for reading should not necessarily be encouraged because the amount of the patient's myopia may differ from the most appropriate add power. Forestalling the use of multifocals by removing glasses for reading may not be helpful in the long run because adaptation to multifocals can be more difficult as the add power increases. Multifocals are also

TABLE 4.1
Summary of Symptoms, Signs, and Recommended Management
of Some Common Binocular Vision Conditions

Condition	Symptoms	Findings	Management
Convergence excess	Eye fatigue and headaches after short periods of reading	Normal distance phoria Esophoria at near High AC/A ratio Low BI vergence at near Low PRA	Plus add to shift near phoria to ortho or low exo or to reduce near eso fixation disparity to zero
Accommodative insufficiency	Blurred near vision, headaches, eyestrain, difficulty reading	High lag of accommodation Low amplitude of accommodation Low PRA finding Slow response on minus side of lens rock	Plus add Subtract 0.25 D from lag on monocular estimate method or Nott retinoscopy, or the add that balances NRA and PRA
Pseudo-convergence insufficiency	Blurred near vision, headaches, eyestrain, difficulty reading	High exo at near secondary to accommodative insufficiency Receded NPC High lag of accommodation NPC improves with an add	Plus add, with power determined as for accommodative insufficiency
Basic exophoria	Eyestrain, headaches, blurred vision, and/or diplopia at distance and near	High exo of approximately the same amount for distance and near AC/A in moderate range BO vergences low at distance and near NRA may be low	Full-time use of full correction of myopia

TABLE 4.1
Continued

Condition	Symptoms	Findings	Management
Divergence excess	Occasional outward eye turn during distance viewing	High exo at distance, normal phoria at near	Full correction for the myopia*
		High AC/A ratio	
Convergence insufficiency	Eyestrain, headaches, drowsiness, and/or diplopia after short periods of reading	Normal distance phoria with high exo at near	Vision therapy to improve BO vergence at near
		Low AC/A ratio	
		Receded NPC	
Accommodative infacility	Intermittent distance blur especially after reading or near work, headaches, eyestrain	Slow response on lens rock monocularly and binocularly	Vision therapy to improve accommodation

AC/A = accommodative convergence–to–accommodation; BI = base in; PRA = positive relative accommodation; NPC = nearpoint convergence; BO = base out; NRA = negative relative accommodation.
*For intermittent exotropia in a young person, overcorrection followed by vision therapy to promote fusion.

preferable to removing glasses for reading for patients with significant amounts of astigmatism or anisometropia.

Glasses or Contact Lenses?

As all practitioners know, a necessary requirement for the wearing of contact lenses is *motivation*; motivation for wearing contact lenses is usually based on a desire to rid oneself of spectacles, either for cosmetic reasons or for sports or other activities in which wearing spectacles is inconvenient or even dangerous. Soft contact lenses, because of the initial comfort that these lenses provide, tend not to require as high a level of motivation—or *determination*—as rigid gas-permeable lenses. Contact lens wear is a good option for myopic patients who are motivated to wear contact lenses, are able and willing to properly care for the lenses, and have adequate corneal physiology to support contact lens wear.

Because motivation for wearing contact lenses is based on a desire to not wear spectacles, it follows that this motivation is usually not likely to be present until the patient is completely dependent on them. In the Houston study of rigid gas-permeable contact lenses for myopia control (Perrigin et al., 1990; Grosvenor et al., 1991a,b), it was found that children who had myopia of no more than approximately 1.00 D, and were therefore not completely dependent on corrective lenses, tended to drop out of the study after just a few weeks or months, whereas children with myopia of 2.00 D or more tended to remain in the study. For children younger than age 11 or 12 years, experience in this study was consistent with that of many practitioners: Although motivation to wear contact lenses may be present, the ability to insert and remove the lenses and to follow instructions in their hygienic care is often lacking. Very young children with very high amounts of myopia or high amounts of myopic anisometropia can be fitted with contact lenses if the parents are capable and motivated to closely monitor lens wear and to insert and remove the lenses as needed (Moore, 1990).

Optical Comparison of Contact Lenses and Spectacles

Optically, contact lenses provide some advantages for the myope—as well as disadvantages—when compared with spectacles.

Field of View

One of the greatest optical advantages of contact lenses as compared with spectacles, no matter what the refractive error may be, is that the visual field of the moving eye—the *dynamic field of view*—is not limited by the frame or by the lens edges. If a contact lens is well centered, has an optic zone larger than the entrance pupil of the eye and moves with the eye, the dynamic field of view is limited only by the ability of the eye to make rotational movements—the *field of fixation.*

Retinal Image Size

When switching from glasses to contact lenses, most myopes do not have to be told that "everything looks bigger" with contact lenses than with glasses. This is true whether the myopia is considered to be axial (which is usually the case) or refractive. For high myopia, the increased retinal image size with contact lenses often results in an improvement in visual acuity.

Anisometropia

Correction of anisometropia with contact lenses results in less aniseikonia than correction with spectacle lenses. This appears to be true whether the origin of the anisometropia is axial or refractive (Bradley et al., 1983; Rabin et al., 1983).

Astigmatism

It will be recalled that a well-centered spherical rigid contact lens—assuming that it does not bend, or flex, while on the eye—eliminates corneal astigmatism but has no effect on internal astigmatism; a well-centered spherical soft contact lens corrects no astigmatism at all. Consequently, the wearer of spherical gas-permeable contact lenses on average has uncorrected against-the-rule astigmatism of approximately –0.50 D, whereas the amount of uncorrected astigmatism experienced by the wearer of spherical soft contact lenses is the total refractive astigmatism of the eye. Toric rigid gas-permeable contact lenses are seldom needed, but toric soft contact lenses should be considered whenever the refractive astigmatism is 0.75 D or 1.00 D or more.

Accommodation

When corrected with a spectacle lens, a myopic eye has an advantage—as compared with an emmetropic eye—that the placement of the correcting lens more than 1 cm in front of the cornea reduces the amount of accommodation needed for near work. Obviously, this advantage is lost when the spectacle lens is replaced with a contact lens. For patients with moderate or high amounts of myopia, the accommodative demand is significantly less with spectacles than with contact lenses (Westheimer, 1962; Benjamin, 1998). For example, the principal plane accommodation required for a person wearing a –5.00 D spectacle lens correction at a vertex distance of 14 mm and viewing an object 40 cm from the spectacle plane is 2.09 D. The principal plane accommodation for that same patient corrected with a contact lenses is 2.41 D (Goss and Eskridge, 1987). The difference in accommodative demand with spectacles and contact lenses increases as the amount of myopia increases. A 10.00 D spectacle lens wearing myope must use only 1.82 D of principal plane accommodation for viewing an object 40 cm from the spectacle plane. With contact lenses, 2.41 D of principal plane accommodation again is needed to view an object 40 cm from the spectacle plane.

For most myopes who are not yet presbyopic, this increased accommodative demand with contact lenses presents no problem. The beginning presbyope who has a moderate or high amount of myopia will have more difficulty reading with contact lenses than with spectacles. A reading addition may be required at a somewhat earlier age with contact lenses than with spectacles. Nonpresbyopes with accommodative disorders may also have more nearpoint difficulties with contact lenses than with glasses.

Case Report

A 40-year-old accountant presented for an eye and vision examination. He reported no problems with his glasses, but he noted that his near vision was blurred with his soft contact lenses. He wore his spectacles for work and for leisure reading, which he did frequently. He wore his contact lenses for his regular jogging, for occasional tennis, and occasionally in the evening. Visual acuities with his spectacles were 20/15 OD and OS at distance and 20/20 OD and OS at near. Nearpoint of accommodation with both eyes viewing and with spectacles in place was approximately 17 cm. The power of his habitual spectacles was –5.50 – 0.50 x 170 OD, –5.50 – 0.25 x 15 OS. The subjective refraction of –5.50 – 0.50 x 173 OD, –5.50 – 0.50 x 10 OS gave distance visual acuities of 20/15 OD and OS. Phorias and fusional vergence ranges were within normal limits. NRA was +2.25 D; PRA was –0.75 D.

Distance visual acuities with his contact lenses were 20/15 OD, OS, OU. Near visual acuities with his contact lenses were 20/30+⅛ OD, 20/30+⅜ OS. Overrefraction with contact lenses in place was +0.25 – 0.25 x 180 OD, +0.25 – 0.25 x 5 OS. Contact lens fit was satisfactory. Ocular health was within normal limits, with myopic temporal crescents present in each eye.

The patient's age, the nearpoint of accommodation almost out to 20 cm, and the low PRA finding indicate approaching presbyopia. He was not yet having difficulty reading with his glasses, but the increased accommodative demand with the contact lenses caused him difficulty seeing at near. No change was made in the spectacle correction, but the patient was educated that bifocals or progressive addition lenses would likely be needed for satisfactory seeing at near in another year or 2. He was also educated concerning the greater near focusing demand with contact lenses than with glasses. He stated that he only rarely read with his contact lenses on, but that it was bothersome enough on those occasions that he decided to get half-eye reading glasses for use with his contact lenses. The patient was advised to return in 6 months for another contact lens check and in 2 years for another complete eye and vision examination, or sooner if he noticed any problems with his vision.

Accommodative Convergence

Because a myope must use more accommodation when wearing contact lenses than when wearing glasses, it follows that more accommodative convergence will be in play during near work. This additional accommodative convergence will bring about a decrease in nearpoint exophoria or an increase in nearpoint esophoria. Except for larger amounts of myopia, the change in the nearpoint phoria is so small as to be negligible. Even for large amounts of myopia, the change in the nearpoint phoria is not large.

The increase in accommodative convergence will depend on the AC/A ratio. For the 5.00 D myope in the example above whose accommodative demand at 40 cm is approximately 2.00 D with glasses but increases to approximately 2.50 D with contact lenses, and for a typical AC/A ratio of 4Δ/D, the additional 0.50 D of accommodative demand would bring about 2Δ of additional accommodative convergence, therefore decreasing a nearpoint exophoria or increasing a nearpoint esophoria by that amount. In a typical convergence insufficiency case, however, in which the patient is essentially orthophoric at distance but has a significant exophoria at near, the AC/A ratio will be very low with the result that the additional accommodative convergence with contact lenses will be negligible.

Lens Centration

The fact that spectacle lenses for nonpresbyopic myopes are usually centered for the distance interpupillary distance (PD) may confer either an advantage or a disadvantage on the wearer in terms of the nearpoint phoria. The prismatic effect at 40 cm can be determined by the use of Prentice's rule, $\Delta = dF$, which states that the induced prismatic effect is equal to the decentration (in cm) times the power of the lens. If a 5 D myope has a nearpoint exophoria of 10Δ and if we assume that lenses are centered for the distance PD and that the eyes converge 4 mm at a distance of 40 cm, the induced prismatic effect (for both eyes) would be

$$0.2 \text{ cm } (-5 \text{ D}) = 2\Delta, \text{ base-in,}$$

which would reduce the nearpoint phoria to 8Δ of exophoria and would also increase the positive fusional vergence reserve by 2Δ. If this patient were to switch to contact lenses—and if we assume that the contact lenses will be well centered on the eyes—the patient would not have the advantage of the 2Δ of induced base-in prism. But for a 2 D myope, the induced base-in prism would be only 0.8Δ, which would probably be negligible.

Practitioners should keep in mind that the nearpoint phoria status can change going from glasses to contact lenses because of this lens centration effect, as well as the accommodative convergence effect noted previously. If the AC/A ratio is moderate, the two effects tend to cancel each other out, but with a high AC/A ratio, the accommodative convergence effect may predominate, and with a low AC/A ratio, the lens centration effect may predominate.

Nearpoint Esophoria

Many young myopic patients are found to be essentially orthophoric at distance but, due to the high AC/A ratio of *convergence excess*, have a significant nearpoint esophoria. In such cases, full-time spectacle lens wear can result in headaches or other symptoms of asthenopia, such that the patient may get into the habit—with or without the advice of the practitioner—of removing the glasses for near work, which of course is the equivalent of wearing a plus add equal to the power of the distance lenses. If the patient is subsequently fitted with contact lenses, which are inconvenient to remove while reading, the lack of the plus add will cause an increase in the nearpoint esophoria, which may result in complaints of asthenopia. (Although the increase in accommodative demand and the change in lens centration may cause minor changes in the nearpoint phoria of a low myope, these are usually negligible when compared with the fact that the contact lenses would be worn for near vision, whereas the spectacle lenses would not.)

When this situation presents itself—that is, when a myope who wears glasses only for distance vision because of a nearpoint esophoria wants to wear contact lenses—the patient should be warned of the possibility of eyestrain during near work unless the contact lenses are removed or unless reading glasses are worn with the contact lenses. The complaint of eyestrain when reading with contact lenses should not automatically be considered a problem in contact lens fit—it may be due to the lack of the plus add at near afforded by taking the glasses off to read.

Soft or Rigid Gas-Permeable Contact Lenses?

As discussed in Chapter 9, rigid gas-permeable contact lenses have been shown to be effective in the control of myopia progression in children and in reducing the existing amount of myopia—orthokeratology—in adults. Continuation of the effect—whether the lenses are used for the control of myopia progression or for orthokeratology—depends, however, on the continued wearing of contact lenses. In orthokeratology, "retainer" lenses may be worn on a part-time basis. Because soft contact lenses do not require such a high degree of motivation, most myopes prefer soft as opposed to rigid lenses if given the choice.

Spectacle Lens Considerations

If spectacle lenses are prescribed, some thought should be given to lens and frame design. The lens reflections that are bothersome in low minus prescriptions can be reduced by the use of antireflection coatings. Antireflection coatings can also be advantageous in high minus lenses in reducing the appearance of the ringlike patterns often seen as a result of reflections from the thick edges of the lenses and because high minus lenses are often made with a fairly flat base curve. Buffing the edges of the lenses also helps to eliminate or minimize these ringlike patterns.

In high minus lenses, steps should be taken to minimize the weight and edge thickness of the lenses (Brooks and Borish, 1979; Fannin and Grosvenor, 1987). Smaller eye sizes and high index materials are helpful in this regard. Measures can also be taken to improve the appearance of thick lens edges. A thick eyewire will better conceal the edge than a thin eyewire or a rimless frame. Hide-a-bevel lens construction helps to conceal the edge by placing the bevel farther forward on the edge of the lens. Rolling and polishing the edge also reduces edge thickness. Edge coating, in which the lens edge is coated to approximately match the frame in color, is another treatment to make the edge less obvious.

The weight and edge thickness of high minus spectacle lenses can be minimized by using lens materials with higher index of refraction values and lower densities. For example, polycarbonate lenses are lighter than CR-39 resin lenses because polycarbonate has a higher index of refraction (1.586 vs. 1.498). Different polyurethane materials have index of refraction values ranging from approximately 1.56 to 1.66. Because high index materials have a high percentage of incident light reflected from them, use of antireflection coating is advisable. Polycarbonate lenses are the appropriate lenses for sports activities and other safety considerations, because they are the most impact-resistant material currently available. Many clinicians routinely use polycarbonate lenses for children because of this characteristic.

In high minus lens prescriptions, accurate PD measurements are important due to the potential of unwanted prismatic effects. For patients with very high amounts of myopia, vertex distance is very important. Frame adjustments that change vertex distance can affect clarity of vision. Vertex distance should be specified on the prescription of very high minus lenses.

Night Myopia and Pseudomyopia

Some patients complain of poor distance vision at night. Under conditions of reduced illumination, accommodation shifts to a position of intermediate distance. That is, for distance viewing, accommodation is greater than necessary. This phenomenon is sometimes referred to as the *dark focus of accommodation*. In one study of college-age subjects, the mean dark focus was 1.52 D, with a standard deviation of 0.77 D and a range of 0 to 4.00 D (Leibowitz and Owens, 1978). As a consequence of the dark focus of accommodation, the retinal image of distant objects is blurred because a small amount of accommodation occurs rather than zero accommodation.

It may be appropriate to correct very low myopia for nighttime vision. For patients who report nighttime distance vision blur and who already wear lenses for myopia, some additional minus may be prescribed for night use only, such as for driving at night. On the basis of work by Owens and Leibowitz (1976) and by Owens et al. (1980), it has been suggested that the additional amount of minus can be derived by performing retinoscopy in a room with all lights off (Goss and Eskridge, 1987). The clinician should, of course, rule out pathologic conditions, such as retinal degenerations, vitamin A deficiencies, glaucoma, or ocular media opacities, as the cause of the poor nighttime seeing (Carr, 1969; Roy, 1989).

Spectacle correction does not improve the vision of former refractive surgery patients who have poor night vision due to increased ocular aberration effects in the peripheral cornea. Such patients may have adequate daytime vision because the pupil diameter is small enough to limit the effects of the aberrations of the eye induced by the surgery.

Other causes of difficulty driving at night include glare from oncoming headlights, poor road design, or unfamiliarity with a given road. Because accommodation does not occur in patients with advanced presbyopia, poor night vision in such patients is not due to the dark focus of accommodation. Older patients may have difficulty driving at night because there is less light transmitted through the eye due to lens opacities and decreased pupil size or because lens opacities may cause light scattering.

If low minus or additional minus is prescribed for night myopia, the patient should be seen in 3–4 weeks after dispensing to see if the symptom of poor night vision has been alleviated. If so, examinations can then be recommended on an annual basis.

☀ CLINICAL PEARL
A low amount of minus lens power or additional minus can improve the vision of a patient's poor distance vision at night due to the dark focus of accommodation.

Pseudomyopia can occur as a result of accommodative excess or accommodative spasm (Stenson and Raskind, 1970; Curtin, 1985; Rutstein et al., 1988). In pseudomyopia, either the manifest refraction is minus while the cycloplegic refraction is plano or plus, or the manifest refraction is more minus than the cycloplegic refraction. The prevalence of pseudomyopia is unknown. In a study by Bannon (1947) conducted on 291 subjects between 10 and 40 years of age who had myopia on manifest refraction, 2.7% had a change of +1.50 D or more under cycloplegia induced by homatropine. If this 2.7% of myopes is then translated into an estimated prevalence in the whole population, it would be less than 1%. Rengstorff (1966) examined the effects of 5% homatropine or 1% cyclopentolate on 122 military recruits. Most subjects were low or medium myopes. The mean effect of the cycloplegic was roughly no change, with one-third of the subjects showing no change, approximately one-third showing a decrease in myopia averaging 0.37 D, and approximately one-third showing an increase in myopia that averaged 0.36 D. Such results suggest a low prevalence of pseudomyopia. Grosvenor et al. (1983, 1984) examined the cycloplegic effect of one drop of 1% cyclopentolate or three to four drops of 1% tropicamide in optometry students. None of the 44 subjects with myopia on manifest refraction had a decrease in myopia of more than 1.00 D with cycloplegia, although a few did decrease in myopia by 0.50 to 1.00 D.

Pseudomyopia is most often found in young persons who do a considerable amount of near work. The patient with pseudomyopia may complain of constant or intermittent distance blur. Asthenopic symptoms may be greater than suggested by test findings. The patient may also complain of blurred distance vision after doing near work. Test findings and observations in pseudomyopia can include some or all of the following: reduced or variable unaided distance visual acuity, apparent low amplitude of accommodation for the patient's age (because part of the amplitude is used in the spasm of accommodation), fluctuations in retinoscopy and subjective refraction, fluctuations in pupil diameter during retinoscopy, more minus on subjective refraction than on retinoscopy, low PRA finding, and high

NRA finding. If some or all of these signs and symptoms are observed, a cycloplegic refraction should be performed to check for pseudomyopia. Pseudomyopia is sometimes associated with high exophoria; it is thought that high exophoria can lead to accommodative excess because accommodative convergence is used to help compensate for the exophoria.

The goal of treatment for pseudomyopia is the relaxation of accommodation. The minus lens power found on manifest refraction should *not* be prescribed. Relaxation of accommodation can be achieved by the use of vision therapy to relax accommodation and improve fusional vergence ranges (Pollack and Grisham, 1980; Apodaca, 1984; Scheiman and Wick, 1994) and by the prescription of near plus adds. In some cases, plus lenses do not eliminate the accommodative excess or spasm by themselves, but can help to prevent future occurrence once accommodation has been relaxed with vision therapy. Some clinicians recommend the therapeutic use of a mild cycloplegic agent to break the accommodative spasm and to aid in the acceptance of the lens prescription obtained under cycloplegic conditions (Rutstein et al., 1988). Trachtman (1978) and Trachtman et al. (1981) presented some case reports in which accommodative biofeedback was reported to reduce pseudomyopia.

Patients should be educated about the nature of pseudomyopia and should be informed that distance vision may be blurry until the accommodative spasm subsides. Patients should be warned against holding reading material too close and should be encouraged to take frequent rest breaks when doing near work. Follow-up checks should be performed every few weeks until the accommodative excess and symptoms have been reduced. At that point, examinations can be provided annually. Many clinicians believe that pseudomyopia is often a precursor to a "real" myopia.

Induced Myopia

Myopia can be induced by certain external agents or by particular internal conditions (Casser Locke, 1987). Patients report distance blur with a time course that is dependent on the nature of the causative factor. There may or may not be other symptoms, again depending on the causative factor.

Various pharmaceutic agents can induce a temporary myopia. For example, cholinergic agonists stimulate accommodation; exposure to them results in pupil constriction along with the induced myopia. Sulfonamides have been reported to induce myopia (Bovino and Marcus, 1982). See Casser Locke (1987) for a listing and discussion of other drugs that can induce myopia.

Another cause of transient induced myopia is the fluctuation in blood sugar levels associated with diabetes mellitus (Goss, 1990). It is thought that this is due to variation in the refractive index of the crystalline lens caused by changes in the blood sugar. Refractive error can change by 1 or 2 D over a matter of hours. Such changes in a patient not diagnosed with diabetes can be an indication for a workup for diabetes. For patients with known diabetes, care should be taken in prescribing spectacles if the diabetes is not under control. It may be advisable to postpone prescribing lenses until the patient no longer notices fluctuations or until the diabetes is under control. One option for temporary use in uncontrolled diabetes is the use of Fresnel lenses.

The treatment of induced myopia is dependent on the cause. Treatment can include recommendations concerning future avoidance of the causative agent or referral for additional testing or treatment. Once the causative factor has been identified, the patient can be informed concerning how long-standing the current episode will be and how to avoid it in the future.

Conclusion and Comments

We have defined myopia correction as the optical compensation for myopia to improve distance visual acuity. Myopia correction is like the correction of any other refractive anomaly in that the goal is to provide clear, comfortable, efficient binocular vision. Factors to consider in deciding whether to prescribe lenses or to change lens powers include the patient's age; amount of myopia; occupational, educational, and recreational visual needs; accommodation and vergence function; and presence of other accompanying conditions. Deciding whether to recommend removing the glasses for near work or whether to prescribe multifocal lenses is dependent on those same factors as well. Myopia correction can be provided in the form of glasses or contact lenses, each of which has its own advantages and disadvantages. Other forms of myopia management are myopia control and myopia reduction, which are discussed in later chapters.

References

Apell RJ. Performance test battery: a very useful tool for prescribing lenses. J Behav Optom 1996;7:7–10.

Apodaca DB. Vision therapy for pseudomyopia. Optom Monthly 1984;75:397–399.

Bannon RE. The use of cycloplegics in refraction. Am J Optom Arch Am Acad Optom 1947;24:513–568.

Benjamin WF. Contact Lenses: Clinical Function and Practical Optics. In WJ Benjamin (ed), Borish's Clinical Refraction. Philadelphia: Saunders, 1998.

Birnbaum MH. Optometric Management of Nearpoint Vision Disorders. Boston: Butterworth–Heinemann, 1993.

Blume AJ. Low-Power Lenses. In JF Amos (ed), Diagnosis and Management in Vision Care. Boston: Butterworths, 1987.

Bovino JA, Marcus JF. The mechanism of transient myopia induced by sulfonamide therapy. Am J Ophthalmol 1982;94:99–102.

Bradley A, Rabin J, Freeman RD. Nonoptical determinants of aniseikonia. Invest Ophthalmol Vis Sci 1983;24:507–512.

Brookman KE. Low Ametropias. In KE Brookman (ed), Refractive Management of Ametropia. Boston: Butterworth–Heinemann, 1996.

Brooks CW, Borish IM. System for Ophthalmic Dispensing. Chicago: Professional Press, 1979;50–51.

Carr RE. The night-blinding disorders. Intern Ophthalmol Clin 1969;9:971–1003.

Casser Locke L. Induced Refractive and Visual Changes. In JF Amos (ed), Diagnosis and Management in Vision Care. Boston: Butterworths, 1987.

Cooper J. Accommodative Dysfunction. In JF Amos (ed), Diagnosis and Management in Vision Care. Boston: Butterworths, 1987.

Cooper J. Intermittent exotropia of the divergence excess type. J Behav Optom 1996;71:67–72.

Cooper J, Duckman R. Convergence insufficiency: incidence, diagnosis, and treatment. J Am Optom Assoc 1978;49:673–680.

Cooper J, Selenow A, Ciuffreda KJ, et al. Reduction of asthenopia in patients with convergence insufficiency after fusional vergence training. Am J Optom Physiol Opt 1983;60:982–989.

Curtin BJ. The Myopias: Basic Science and Clinical Management. Philadelphia: Harper & Row, 1985;455–467.

Daum KM. Accommodative dysfunction. Doc Ophthalmol 1983a;55:177–198.

Daum KM. Accommodative insufficiency. Am J Optom Physiol Opt 1983b; 60:352–359.

Daum KM. Characteristics of exodeviations. II. Changes with treatment with orthoptics. Am J Optom Physiol Opt 1986;63:244–251.

Daum KM. Accommodative Response. In JB Eskridge, JF Amos, JD Bartlett (eds), Clinical Procedures in Optometry. Philadelphia: Lippincott, 1991.

Fannin TE, Grosvenor T. Clinical Optics. Boston: Butterworths, 1987;382–388.

Flax N. Management of divergence excess intermittent exotropia. J Behav Optom 1996;71:66, 72, 73.

Goss DA. Refractive Changes in Diabetes. In DA Goss, LL Edmondson (eds), Eye and Vision Conditions in the American Indian. Yukon, OK: Pueblo Publishing, 1990;53–59.

Goss DA. Fixation Disparity. In JB Eskridge, JF Amos, JD Bartlett (eds), Clinical Procedures in Optometry. Philadelphia: Lippincott, 1991.

Goss DA. Ocular Accommodation, Convergence, and Fixation Disparity: A Manual of Clinical Analysis (2nd ed). Boston: Butterworth–Heinemann, 1995.

Goss DA. Determining the optimal nearpoint plus prescription based on case types and examination test results. J Behav Optom 1996a;7:6, 10, 11.

Goss DA. Myopia. In KE Brookman (ed), Refractive Management of Ametropia. Boston: Butterworth–Heinemann, 1996b.

Goss DA, Eskridge JB. Myopia. In JF Amos (ed), Diagnosis and Management in Vision Care. Boston: Butterworths, 1987.

Goss DA, Grosvenor T. Reliability of refraction: a literature review. J Am Optom Assoc 1996;67:619–630.

Goss DA, Grosvenor TP, Keller JT, et al. Optometric Clinical Practice Guideline—Care of the Patient with Myopia. St. Louis: American Optometric Association, 1998.

Griffin JR. Efficacy of vision therapy for nonstrabismic vergence anomalies. Am J Optom Physiol Opt 1987;64:411–414.

Griffin JR, Grisham JD. Binocular Anomalies: Diagnosis and Vision Therapy (3rd ed). Boston: Butterworth–Heinemann, 1995;89–90.

Grisham JD. Visual therapy results for convergence insufficiency: a literature review. Am J Optom Physiol Opt 1988;65:448–454.

Grosvenor T. Primary Care Optometry—Anomalies of Refraction and Binocular Vision (3rd ed). Boston: Butterworth–Heinemann, 1996;361–368, 434–435.

Grosvenor T, Perrigin D, Perrigin J, Quintero S. Rigid gas-permeable contact lenses for myopia control. Optom Vis Sci 1991a;68:385–389.

Grosvenor T, Perrigin D, Perrigin J, Quintero S. Do gas permeable contact lenses control the progression of myopia? Cont Lens Spectrum 1991b;6:29–35.

Grosvenor T, Perrigin D, Perrigin J, et al. A comparison of cycloplegic and noncycloplegic refractive findings on a group of young adults. Texas Optom 1983;(Dec):7–8; and 1984;(Jan):8–11.

Gwiazda J, Thorn F, Bauer J, Held R. Emmetropization and the progression of manifest refraction in children followed from infancy to puberty. Clin Vis Sci 1993;8:337–344.

Haynes HM. Clinical approaches to nearpoint power determination. Am J Optom Physiol Opt 1985;62:375–385.

Kurtz D. Presbyopia. In KE Brookman (ed), Refractive Management of Ametropia. Boston: Butterworth–Heinemann, 1996.

Leibowitz HW, Owens DA. New evidence for the intermediate position of relaxed accommodation. Doc Ophthalmol 1978;46:133–147.

Moore BD. Contact Lens Problems and Management in Infants, Toddlers, and Preschool Children. In MM Scheiman (ed), Problems in Optometry: Pediatric Optometry. Philadelphia: Lippincott, 1990;2:365–393.

Newman JM. Analysis, Interpretation, and Prescription for the Ametropias and Heterophorias. In WJ Benjamin (ed), Borish's Clinical Refraction. Philadelphia: Saunders, 1998.

Owens DA, Leibowitz HW. Night myopia: cause and a possible basis for amelioration. Am J Optom Physiol Opt 1976;53:709–717.

Owens DA, Mohindra I, Held R. The effectiveness of a retinoscope beam as an accommodative stimulus. Invest Ophthalmol Vis Sci 1980;19:942–949.

Patorgis CJ. Presbyopia. In JF Amos (ed), Diagnosis and Management Vision Care. Boston: Butterworths, 1987.

Perrigin J, Perrigin D, Quintero S, Grosvenor T. Silicone-acrylate contact lenses for myopia control: 3-year results. Optom Vis Sci 1990;67:764–769.

Pollack SL, Grisham JD. Orthoptics for pseudomyopia. Rev Optom 1980;117:35–38.

Rabin J, Bradley A, Freeman RD. On the relation between aniseikonia and axial anisometropia. Am J Optom Physiol Opt 1983;60:553–558.

Rengstorff RH. Observed effects of cycloplegia on refractive findings. J Am Optom Assoc 1966;37:360.

Richman JE, Cron MT. Guide to Vision Therapy. South Bend, IN: Bernell Corporation, 1987;17–18.

Rouse MW. Management of binocular anomalies: efficacy of vision therapy in the treatment of accommodative disorders. Am J Optom Physiol Opt 1987;64: 415–420.

Rouse MW, London R, Allen DC. An evaluation of the monocular estimate method of dynamic retinoscopy. Am J Optom Physiol Opt 1982;59:234–239.

Roy FH. Ocular Differential Diagnosis (4th ed). Philadelphia: Lea & Febiger, 1989;691–693.

Rutstein RP, Daum KM. Anomalies of Binocular Vision: Diagnosis and Management. St. Louis: Mosby, 1998;162–163.

Rutstein RP, Daum KM, Amos JF. Accommodative spasm: a study of 17 cases. J Am Optom Assoc 1988;59:527–538.

Saladin JJ. Phorometry and stereopsis. In WJ Benjamin (ed), Borish's Clinical Refraction. Philadelphia: Saunders, 1998.

Scheiman M, Wick B. Clinical Management of Binocular Vision: Heterophoric, Accommodative, and Eye Movement Disorders. Philadelphia: Lippincott, 1994.

Stenson SM, Raskind RH. Pseudomyopia: etiology, mechanisms, and therapy. J Pediatr Ophthalmol 1970;7:110–115.

Steward JM, Cole BL, Pettit JL. Visual difficulty driving at night. Aust J Optom 1983;66:20–24.

Suchoff IB, Petito GT. The efficacy of visual therapy accommodative disorders and non–strabismic anomalies of binocular vision. J Am Optom Assoc 1986;57: 119–125.

Trachtman JN. Biofeedback of accommodation to reduce functional myopia: a case report. Am J Optom Physiol Opt 1978;55:400–406.

Trachtman JN, Giambalvo V, Feldman J. Biofeedback of accommodation to reduce functional myopia. Biofeedback Self Regul 1981;6:547–564.

Westheimer G. The visual world of the new contact lens wearer. J Am Optom Assoc 1962;34:135–138.

Wick BC. Horizontal deviations. In JF Amos (ed), Diagnosis and Management in Vision Care. Boston: Butterworths, 1987.

PART **II**

Methods of Myopia Control and Reduction

CHAPTER 5

Vision Therapy

Vision therapy (or vision training) has sometimes been suggested as a means of either lowering the rate of myopia progression (myopia control) or reducing the amount of existing myopia (myopia reduction). Many different vision therapy techniques have been proposed. Unfortunately, there is a paucity of good studies evaluating the effectiveness of vision therapy in myopia control or myopia reduction. What is indisputable from several studies is that a wide variety of methods have been successful in improving unaided visual acuity in patients with myopia, even though the amount of myopia may not be reduced (e.g., Rowe, 1947; Bateman, 1948; Preble, 1948; Kennedy, 1951; Zaikova et al., 1978; Collins et al., 1981, 1982; Balliett et al., 1982; Matson et al., 1983; Berman et al., 1985; and other articles and book chapters discussed below). Explanations suggested for improved, unaided acuity include an increased ability to interpret blurred images, practice effects, psychological factors, and changes in tear distribution, but the correct reason is unknown (Bannon, 1942; Lancaster, 1944; Birnbaum, 1993).

Published studies on vision therapy for myopia reduction are discussed in this chapter. Also discussed are some vision therapy programs that have been proposed for myopia control.

The Baltimore Project

A well-publicized study on the effects of visual training on myopia is the Baltimore project, conducted from September 1943 to December 1943 to determine whether visual training could reduce myopia. The 103 subjects who completed the training ranged in age from 9 to 32 years, and averaged 25 training sessions. Subjects had myopia that ranged from –0.50 to –9.00 D, although there was one subject who had antimetropia. Optometrists and technicians did the training, although details of the training procedures were not published. An optometric team sponsored by the American

Optometric Association and an ophthalmologic team from the Wilmer Eye Institute evaluated the outcome of the training. Measurements included visual acuity with letters, numbers, Landolt Cs, and tumbling Es, as well as cycloplegic retinoscopy. Several reports summarized the results of the study (Woods, 1945; Ewalt, 1946; Shepard, 1946; Hackman, 1947; Betts, 1947; Hildreth, 1947). Most subjects had an improvement in unaided visual acuity. The improvement in acuity averaged approximately two lines of letters. Changes in cycloplegic retinoscopy for 67 of the subjects were discussed in the article written by Woods (1945). Some subjects showed increases in myopia and some showed decreases, but there did not appear to be an overall trend toward myopia reduction.

Biofeedback Studies

A few publications have reported the use of biofeedback as a potential means of reducing myopia. Most of these studies have used the commercially available Accommotrac Vision Trainer (Biofeedback, Inc., Brooklyn Heights, NY), which couples an infrared optometer with auditory biofeedback. This device was developed by Trachtman (1987) and is used to decrease accommodation levels.

The first case report of biofeedback for myopia appears to have been published by Trachtman (1978). A 30-year-old man had seven biofeedback training sessions totaling 34 minutes. Unaided visual acuity improved from 20/50-2 OD, 20/50-2 OS to 20/30+2 OD, 20/30-2 OS. The minus in the subjective refraction decreased from –0.75 –0.50 x 90 OD, –0.75 sph OS, to plano sph OD, –0.25 sph OS. Retinoscopy findings showed little difference with training (–0.75 –0.75 x 100 OD, –1.25 –0.75 x 90 OS before training and –1.00 sph OD, –1.25 sph OS after training).

Trachtman et al. (1981) published three case reports of the biofeedback training of three males in their early thirties. Each had spherical refractive errors of –0.25 to –0.75 D, onset of myopia in the late teens or early 20s, a history of extensive near work, high negative relative accommodation test findings, and a difference in amount of myopia on retinoscopy and subjective refraction. It was presumed that the myopia was due to ciliary muscle spasm. Two of the three patients had slight improvements in unaided visual acuity from 20/25+ or 20/20– to 20/20– or 20/20+. One patient showed an improvement in visual acuity from 20/70-2 OD, 20/100-2 OS to 20/40+2 OD, 20/20-1 OS. In five of the eyes, the minus in the subjective refraction decreased by at least 0.25 D.

Trachtman (1990) presented data on biofeedback training for myopia reduction on 84 patients using the Accommotrac Vision Trainer from a private practice. The median age of the patients was 27.5 years, with a range of 8–62 years. The number of training sessions varied from patient to patient, with a median of eight sessions, and a range of 1–29 sessions. The training sessions lasted 1 hour, with rest periods alternating with testing and training periods. Later in the training program, there was home training, which, it was hoped, would generalize biofeedback training to the everyday environment. Decreases in minus power in the patient's habitual spectacle correction were prescribed, and in some cases plus for near vision was used. Refractive error measurements were subjective refractions to the minimum minus power yielding 20/20 visual acuity. The median unaided visual acuity before training was 20/187.5 (range, 20/20 to 20/1000). After training, the median acuity was 20/30 (range, 20/15 to 20/200). The median pretraining refractive correction was –2.37 D (range, –0.25 to –11.50 D). After training, the median refractive correction was –0.75 D (range, plano to –7.00 D). This study would have been improved if objective refractive data were also available, because the outcome of a subjective procedure with an acuity criterion could have been affected by improvements in visual acuity exclusive of refractive change.

Trachtman (1990) also reported a compilation of 240 case histories of Accommotrac training from 11 optometry practices and one ophthalmology practice. There was an average of 11 training sessions per subject. The median pretraining visual acuity was 20/200. The median post-training visual acuity was 20/30. The median change in refractive correction was +0.87 D, with a range of 0 to +4.75 D. Methods for determining refractive correction were not stated.

Other published studies on the use of biofeedback for myopia reduction have not shown results as successful as Trachtman's (1990). Gallaway et al. (1987) tested the Accommotrac Vision Trainer on 11 subjects with myopia of 4 D or less. Ten of the subjects were optometry students who ranged in age from 23 to 33 years. The other subject was a 42-year-old faculty member. Eight subjects completed at least 12 biofeedback training sessions. One subject completed eight sessions. Seven of these nine subjects had improvements in unaided visual acuity. The largest improvement in visual acuity was from 20/110 to 20/26. Improvements in acuity were maintained during follow-up periods of a few weeks. The improvements in unaided visual acuity were not accompanied by reductions in myopia. The mean change in spherical equivalent refractive error measured by autorefraction was –0.10 D. Three subjects reported a significant monocular diplopia or triplopia.

Koslowe et al. (1991) tested the Accommotrac Vision Trainer on a treatment group of nine female and six male subjects, whose average age was 20 (range, 10–40 years) and whose average refractive error was –4.50 D of myopia (range, –1.00 to –9.25 D). A control group of seven females and eight males were an average age of 20.3 years. The treatment group had 10 biofeedback training sessions. Koslowe et al. reported that there was no difference in the change in unaided visual acuity, retinoscopy, or subjective refraction between the treatment and control groups.

Angi et al. (1996) studied the effects of biofeedback training with a device manufactured in Italy, the Visual Training System (Epsilon Srl, Florence, Italy). Like the Accommotrac, it links an infrared optometer with an auditory feedback system. Twenty-one secondary school girls were trained. Subject inclusion criteria were corrected decimal visual acuity of 1.0 in both eyes, spherical cycloplegic refractive error of less than –3.50 D myopia, anisometropia and astigmatism of less than 1.25 D, presence of stereopsis, and no ocular or systemic disease. The mean age of the subjects was 17.4 years. Refractive errors were determined by autorefraction under manifest conditions and under cyclopentolate cycloplegia. Right eye spherical refractive error was –1.20 D (SD = 0.9) before training and –1.29 D (SD = 1.0) a little more than a year after training. Left eye auto refraction was –1.29 D (SD = 1.0) before training and –1.47 D (SD = 1.0) a year after training. The difference in right eye refraction was not statistically significant, but the difference in left eye refractive error was significant (p <.01). Right eye unaided decimal visual acuity was 0.42 before training and 0.58 a little more than a year after the training was completed. Left eye acuity was 0.40 before training and 0.51 after training. The unaided visual acuities were significantly better after training for both right eyes (p <.01) and left eyes (p <.03). A control group of untreated myopes and a group of emmetropes and hyperopes did not show an improvement in unaided visual acuity. Psychological assessment showed that the treated myopes had "an improved subjective perception of psychological well-being."

Angi et al. (1996) also noted that their treated subjects often reported a sensation of warmth and increased eye volume after training. Subjects also occasionally reported monocular diplopia with the perception of a central blurred image accompanied by a clearer image alongside. Angi et al. observed bilateral mydriasis when the feedback sounds associated with decreased accommodation were occurring. Some subjects were able to recall that sound sensation while being tested with an autorefractor. The recollection of the sound resulted in bilateral mydriasis, but an *increase* in myopia. These changes did not occur under cycloplegia. None of the subjects were able to decrease minus while recalling the feedback sound. Angi et al. speculated that an increase in choroidal blood flow at the macula may have been responsible for these seemingly paradoxical results. Whatever the correct explanation may be, these observations demonstrate that we have much yet to learn about biofeedback for myopia.

Barton et al. (in preparation) trained seven subjects with the Accommotrac Vision Trainer. The subjects had 11–14 training sessions over an 8- to 9-week period. Subjects ranged in age from 12.2 to 40.7 years (mean age, 26.3 years). Unaided distance visual acuity improved from 20/115 to 20/61 in the right eye, and from 20/144 to 20/56 in the left eye. The changes were statistically significant by Wilcoxon signed ranks test (p <.02 for each eye). The mean manifest subjective refraction changed from –4.02 to –3.72 D in the right eye and from –4.21 to –3.91 D in the left eye. The mean change in refractive error was +0.30 D in each eye. The mean changes in subjective refraction just missed being statistically significant by paired t-test (p <.1 for each eye).

In an extensive review of study results and theoretical issues associated with biofeedback for myopia, Gilmartin et al. (1991) concluded that additional studies are needed "before accommodation biofeedback can qualify as an established method of clinical treatment of myopia." Among their suggestions for further study was the recommendation that an adequate theoretical framework for the effects of biofeedback should be correlated with the current knowledge concerning the etiology of myopia. One could also ask whether biofeedback might be better suited for myopia control than for myopia reduction. To date, studies with biofeedback have been designed to decrease accommodation. As discussed in Chapter 2 and in other more extensive reviews (Goss and Zhai, 1994; Ong and Ciuffreda, 1997), myopia appears to be associated with decreased accommodation for near. Perhaps a biofeedback regimen that decreases accommodation for distance and increases accommodation for near to reduce retinal defocus for near objects could be developed for myopia control, rather than for myopia reduction.

Studies on Various Behavioral Training Methods

A few studies have involved training methods that did not incorporate lenses or prisms and therefore did not change the stimuli to accommodation and vergence.

Berens et al. (1957) studied the effects of a tachistoscopic training procedure on myopia. The procedure involved exposure of groups of digits, with the number of digits being shown increasing and exposure time decreasing as training progressed. Subjects with lower amounts of myopia were encouraged to do the training without their spectacles and to move as far away from the screen as possible, moving back gradually to 20 feet. A total of 140 subjects, ages 6–47 years, participated in the study. The treatment group consisted of 80 persons, with a mean age of 22.75 years (SD = 10.01) and an average refractive error of –2.27 D (SD = 1.47). In the control group, there were 60 persons, with a mean age of 22.32 years (SD = 9.71), and a mean refraction equal to –2.31 D (SD = 1.05). Treatment group subjects attended 30-minute group training sessions, three times a week for 10 weeks. Changes in mean unaided visual acuity in the experimental group were from 20/125 to 20/77 monocularly and from 20/98 to 20/63 binocularly. In the control group, the change was from 20/115 to 20/157 monocularly and from 20/97 to 20/131 binocularly. Both groups had statistically significant changes in refractive error measured by retinoscopy. The treatment group had a decrease in myopia of +0.22 D. The control group had an increase in myopia of –0.29 D. Therefore, it appears that this relatively simple training procedure results in a slight reduction in myopia.

Giddings and Lanyon (1974) showed that positive reinforcement on a visual acuity task could produce short-term decreases in myopia. The subjects were 60 male volunteers from introductory psychology classes at the University of Pittsburgh. Their refractive corrections were between –1.00

and –5.00 D, with less than 1.00 D of astigmatism. Subjects were randomly assigned to one of three treatment groups: positive reinforcement, noncontingent reinforcement, and control. The training procedure started by having the subjects sit in a comfortable chair and listen to an 11-minute instructional tape on physical relaxation. Then the subjects viewed a series of slides, each of which had four rings, one with an opening like a Landolt C. The subjects reported which of the rings was the one with the opening. The positive reinforcement group subjects were told when they were correct. The noncontingent reinforcement groups received verbal encouragement on a random basis unrelated to whether their response was correct. The control group received no verbal response from the experimenter. All three groups showed an improvement in visual acuity. The positive reinforcement group had less myopia at the end of the training period than at the beginning as measured by retinoscopy. The exact amount of change was not given, but it was 0.22 D more than the change in the control group and 0.20 D more than the change in the noncontingent reinforcement group.

Rosen et al. (1984) used a training program similar to that of Giddings and Lanyon (1974), but over a 6-week period. Twenty-nine subjects, ages 19–47 years, were assigned to one of three groups: behavioral training plus feedback group (n = 10), behavioral training only (n = 10), and no treatment control group (n = 9). The behavioral training consisted of instructions for avoiding eyestrain, for eye relaxation massage techniques, for "a brief eye exercise regimen to be performed several times daily," and for "practicing accommodation by fixating on targets at increasing distances." No additional details were provided on these behavioral training procedures. The two treatment groups also were trained on a Landolt ring discrimination task such as that used by Giddings and Lanyon. The behavioral-training-plus-feedback group were told when they made correct responses, whereas the behavioral-training-only group was not.

Rosen et al. (1984) reported that the behavioral-training-plus-feedback group had improvements in acuity in both eyes: from 20/128 to 20/65 in the right eye and 20/95 to 20/60 in the left eye. The improvements in acuity in the behavioral-training-only group were from 20/133 to 20/95 in the right eye and from 20/125 to 20/59 in the left eye. The changes in acuity in the treatment groups were significantly different from the changes in the control group (20/133 to 20/133 in the right eye and 20/140 to 20/128 in the left eye). In the behavioral-training-plus-feedback group, refractive error decreased from –2.30 D to –2.18 D in the right eye and –2.33 D to –2.05 D in the left eye. Refractive error changes in the behavioral-training-only group were from –2.35 D to –1.98 D in the right eye and from –2.25 D to –2.20 D in the left eye. Refractive changes were negligible in the control group: from –2.69 D to –2.69 D in the right eye and from –2.81 D to –2.86 D in the left eye. There appeared to be a trend toward decreased myopia of approximately a quarter diopter in the two treatment groups, but analysis of variance did not show a statistically significant change.

Leber and Wilson (1993) reported on the results of seven subjects on a computer-based training program. Four letters were displayed on a computer screen. Subjects used a keyboard-entry system to respond to each set of letters, entering what they believed the letters to be. If a letter or letters were identified incorrectly, the correct letters were displayed in larger size. If all letters were identified correctly, a new set of smaller letters was displayed. The seven subjects were males, ages 19–23 years. Each subject underwent five 1-hour training sessions. Six of the subjects sat 20 feet from the computer screen during training. One subject initially had 20/250 unaided visual acuity, and sat 10 feet from the computer screen. Of seven right eyes, there was no improvement in unaided visual acuity in two eyes, and an improvement of one line in five eyes. For the seven left eyes, there was no improvement in two eyes, one-line improvement in three eyes, and two-line improvement in two eyes. Refractive error remained unchanged in five right eyes and changed by +0.25 D in two right eyes. Myopia remained unchanged in one left eye, and decreased by +0.25 D in six left eyes. The method of refractive error measurement was not stated.

Each of the training methods in the four studies resulted in significantly improved unaided visual acuities. Each of the studies also showed a mean myopia reduction of approximately +0.25 D.

Vision Therapy Programs for Myopia Control

Some of the vision training programs for myopia control that have been described in the optometric literature are summarized below. Many aspects of these programs appear to be logical approaches to the problem, but unfortunately there do not appear to be any data on their efficacy.

Friedman

Friedman (1981) described a program for myopia control that consists of minimum use of full-correction minus lenses, use of plus power training lenses, adherence to guidelines concerning use of the eyes ("visuobehavioral guidelines"), and a short, intensive vision training program. The visuobehavioral guidelines regarding reading are as follows: Do not read under stressful conditions. Do not read very small print or poor-quality print. Avoid reading in dim light, in cramped postures, or in moving vehicles. Take regular distance-viewing breaks during reading.

Some of the visuobehavioral guidelines for daily viewing are as follows: Avoid intensive visual concentration. View objects in a relaxed manner. Do not strain to see. Do not rigidly maintain eye position. Increase awareness of peripheral visual space. Several times a day, look at a faraway scene or close your eyes and visualize a distant relaxing outdoor view.

The training program Friedman advocated consists of 10–12 weekly 1-hour in-office training sessions and 30 minutes of daily home training. The primary goals of the training are to help the patient learn voluntary control of accommodation, to learn self-awareness of accommodative function, and to improve accommodation and convergence function. The training procedures include teaching the patients to be able to alternately clear or blur their vision when looking through lenses of various powers, thus learning better awareness and control of accommodation. The training program also includes various standard accommodation, vergence, and anti-suppression training techniques such as cheiroscopes, monocular and binocular lens rock accommodative facility training, Brock string, aperture rule, vectograph slides, and so on.

Friedman stated that he believed this program was the most effective in controlling myopia for patients with adult-onset myopia and the least effective for patients younger than age 12. He also suggested that patients with significant accommodation and vergence dysfunctions were more likely to have their myopia controlled when accommodation and vergence skills are improved. Unfortunately, Friedman (1981) did not present any data.

Birnbaum

Birnbaum (1993) advocated a vision therapy program composed of near-point plus lens additions, "visual hygiene" recommendations concerning near work, and training to improve accommodation and vergence skills for incipient and progressing myopia. For "visual hygiene," patients are advised to read in a relaxed manner, with good posture in a comfortable chair, and with proper, glare-free lighting. Patients are told to take short breaks during near work activities and to frequently look out at distant objects. Patients who are intense readers are advised to get up and walk around for approximately a minute after each 10–15 minutes of reading. The working distance for near work should be about the distance from the elbow to the second knuckle. For reading or computer work, the patient is advised to maintain a relaxed attitude, with application of relaxation and peripheral awareness procedures to recognize and reduce body tension (Birnbaum, 1990). Birnbaum (1984, 1985) stated that stress reduction is important because the sympathetic nervous system arousal associated with stress is likely to cause a decrease in accommodation. He suggested that repeated exposure to stress from heavy near work demands leads to overconvergence and that myopia is an adaptation to avoid the nearpoint stress of decreased accommodation and overconvergence.

The training procedures recommended by Birnbaum (1993) are monocular and binocular accommodative facility training, fusional vergence range extension with emphasis on base-in ranges, accommodation relaxation, and plus acceptance procedures. Fusional vergence ranges can be enhanced beyond a basic level by training base-out ranges through plus lens additions and by training base-in ranges through minus adds, sometimes referred to as *BOP-BIM training*.

Sherman and Press

Sherman and Press (1997), like Birnbaum (1984, 1985, 1993), viewed myopia as an adaptation to visual stress, and they incorporated several of Birnbaum's concepts in their recommendations for myopia control. Sherman and Press recommended development of greater accommodation relaxation capability, expansion of base-in fusional vergence ranges, use of mental imagery to visualize distant objects, reduction of attentional intensity, reduction of general stress, and expansion of peripheral awareness. Sherman and Press also made recommendations similar to Birnbaum's concerning proper working distance, posture, and ergonomics for reading and computer work. They recommended nearpoint plus lens additions when indicated by test findings, oculomotor therapy if eye movement skills are deficient, and accommodative facility training.

☀ **CLINICAL PEARL**

It is clear that a variety of training programs improve unaided visual acuity in myopia. It is less clear that these training programs can reduce myopia by a significant amount. Based on what we know about myopia etiology, it may be possible to design therapy programs to control myopia progression.

Conclusion and Comments

Although 50 years apart, Stoddard (1942) and Birnbaum (1993) both suggested that myopia could be reduced by no more than approximately 0.75 D. Citing master's thesis research done at the University of California in 1941 by Chance, Stoddard noted that the patients who showed reductions in myopia with training are those who had more myopia under manifest conditions than under cycloplegic conditions. In four studies on behavioral training techniques treatment, there were mean decreases in myopia of approximately a quarter diopter. Results of studies on biofeedback for myopia reduction have been variable.

To date, there do not appear to be any published studies on vision therapy for myopia control. The three vision therapy programs summarized in this chapter are similar. In the absence of data showing their efficacy, we can ask whether such procedures could affect the various factors thought to contribute to myopia. As discussed in Chapter 2, a prominent contemporary theory is that retinal image defocus plays a role in myopia development. Thus, procedures that improve accommodative accuracy might be expected to control myopia. It seems possible that vision-training procedures for better accommodative function and better perception of distance cues for control of accommodation could contribute to myopia control. The same could be said about behavioral recommendations concerning avoidance of stress and other factors that might affect autonomic nervous system function and thus accommodation, or concerning avoidance of situations that might lead to accommodative fatigue or to accommodative inaccuracy. This is certainly an area that needs further development and investigation.

References

Angi MR, Caucci S, Pilotto E, et al. Changes in myopia, visual acuity, and psychological distress after biofeedback visual training. Optom Vis Sci 1996;73:35–42.

Balliett R, Clay A, Blood K. The training of visual acuity in myopia. J Am Optom Assoc 1982;53:719–724.

Bannon RE. On the reduction of myopia. Columbia Optom 1942;16(63):2,3,6.

Barton LG, Young TW, Goss DA. Training voluntary accommodation in myopic patients with the Accommotrac Vision Trainer, manuscript in preparation.

Bateman E. Comment on the treatment of myopia. Am J Optom Arch Am Acad Optom 1948;25:241–242.

Berens C, Girard LJ, Fonda G, Sells SB. Effects of tachistoscopic training on visual functions in myopic patients. Am J Ophthalmol 1957;44:25–48.

Berman PE, Levinger SI, Massoth NA, et al. The effectiveness of biofeedback visual training as a viable method of treatment and reduction of myopia. J Optom Vis Dev 1985;16:17, 19–21.

Betts EA. An evaluation of the Baltimore myopia control project. Part A: experimental procedures. J Am Optom Assoc 1947;18:481–485.

Birnbaum MH. Nearpoint visual stress: a physiological model. J Am Optom Assoc 1984;55:825–835.

Birnbaum MH. Nearpoint visual stress: clinical implications. J Am Optom Assoc 1985;56:480–490.

Birnbaum MH. The use of stress reduction concepts and techniques in vision therapy. J Behav Optom 1990;1:3–7.

Birnbaum MH. Optometric Management of Nearpoint Vision Disorders. Boston: Butterworth–Heinemann, 1993;303–309.

Collins FJ, Epstein LH, Hannay HJ. A component analysis of operant training program for improving visual acuity in myopic students. Behav Ther 1981;12:692–701.

Collins FL, Ricci JA, Burkett PA. Behavioral training for myopia: long-term maintenance of improved acuity. Behav Res Ther 1982;19:265–268.

Ewalt HW Jr. The Baltimore myopia control project. J Am Optom Assoc 1946;17:167–185.

Friedman E. Vision training program for myopia management. Am J Optom Physiol Opt 1981;58:546–553.

Gallaway M, Pearl SM, Winkelstein AM, Scheiman M. Biofeedback training of visual acuity and myopia: a pilot study. Am J Optom Physiol Opt 1987;64:62–71.

Giddings JW, Lanyon RI. Effect of reinforcement of visual acuity in myopic adults. Am J Optom Physiol Opt 1974;51:181–188.

Gilmartin B, Gray LS, Winn B. The amelioration of myopia using biofeedback of accommodation: a review. Ophthal Physiol Opt 1991;11:304–313.

Goss DA, Zhai H. Clinical and laboratory investigations on the relationship of accommodation and convergence function with refractive error—a literature review. Doc Ophthalmol 1994;86:349–380.

Hackman RB. An evaluation of the Baltimore myopia project. Part B: statistical procedure. J Am Optom Assoc 1947;18:416–426.

Hildreth HR, Meinberg WH, Milder B, et al. The effect of visual training on existing myopia. Trans Am Acad Ophthalmol Otolaryngol 1947;51:260–277.

Kennedy JR. A case of an uncorrected child myope showing progression in presence of visual training. Am J Optom Arch Am Acad Optom 1951;28:642–644.

Koslowe KC, Spierer A, Rosner M, Belkin M. Evaluation of Accommotrac biofeedback training for myopia control. Optom Vis Sci 1991;68:338–343.

Lancaster WB. Present status of eye exercises for improvement of visual functions. Arch Ophthalmol 1944;32:167–172.

Leber L, Wilson TA. Myopia reduction training with a computer-based behavioral technique: a preliminary report. J Behav Optom 1993;4:87–90,92.

Matson JL, Helsel WJ, LaGrow SJ. Training visual efficiency in myopic persons. Behav Res Ther 1983;21:115–118.

Ong E, Ciuffreda KJ. Accommodation, Nearwork, and Myopia. Santa Ana, CA: Optometric Extension Program, 1997.

Preble D. Visual training in myopia—a case report. Am J Optom Arch Am Acad Optom 1948;25:545–547.

Rosen RC, Schiffman HR, Meyers H. Behavioral treatment of myopia: refractive error and acuity changes in relation to axial length and intraocular pressure. Am J Optom Physiol Opt 1984;61:100–105.

Rowe AJ. Orthoptic training to improve the visual acuity of a myope—a case report. Am J Optom Arch Am Acad Optom 1947;24:494.

Shepard CF. The Baltimore project. Optom Weekly 1946;37:133–135.

Sherman A, Press LJ. Myopia Control Therapy. In LJ Press (ed), Applied Concepts in Vision Therapy. St. Louis: Mosby, 1997;298–309.

Stoddard KB. Physiological limitations on the functional production and elimination of ametropia. Am J Optom Arch Am Acad Optom 1942;19:112–118.

Trachtman JN. Biofeedback of accommodation to reduce functional myopia: a case report. Am J Optom Physiol Opt 1978;55:400–406.

Trachtman JN. Biofeedback of accommodation to reduce myopia: a review. Am J Optom Physiol Opt 1987;64:639–643.

Trachtman JN. The Etiology of Vision Disorders: A Neuroscience Model. Santa Ana, California: Optometric Extension Program, 1990;73–83.

Trachtman JN, Giambalvo V, Feldman J. Biofeedback of accommodation to reduce functional myopia. Biofeedback Self-Regulation 1981;6:547–562.

Woods AC. Report from the Wilmer Institute on the results obtained in the treatment of myopia by visual training. Trans Am Acad Ophthalmol Otolaryngol 1945;50:37–65.

Zaikova MV, Burdelova SF, Stronskaia VA, Parygina NP. Experience with the treatment of myopia at a specialized pioneer camp. Vestn Oftalmol 1978;(1): 40–42.

CHAPTER 6

Control with Added Plus Power for Near Work

From a theoretical standpoint, added lens power for near work appears to be a reasonable approach to myopia control. One theory of the etiology of myopia (see Chapter 2) involves mechanical effects on the eye due to accommodation levels being too high. Another theory involves the defocus effects of accommodative responses being too low for the dioptric accommodative stimulus. In either case, added plus at near could be a viable option for the prevention or control. In the former theory (accommodation levels being too high), the accommodative stimulus could be reduced by the use of nearpoint plus additions, thereby reducing the amount of accommodation occurring. In the latter theory (accommodative response being less than the accommodative stimulus, therefore producing a defocus), the amount of defocus of the retinal image could be reduced by the use of additional plus lens power for near viewing. Added plus in the form of bifocal lenses has been studied extensively. Myopia control effects of added plus by means of removing one's glasses for near work, undercorrection of myopia, or progressive addition lenses have received limited study.

Bifocals

Studies investigating the effect of bifocals on childhood myopia progression have included studies using a retrospective examination of private practice patient records, as well as prospective longitudinal studies performed in clinics. Results of different studies have been variable, which could be explained by a number of factors, one of which may be that the effectiveness of bifocal control of myopia may depend on patient characteristics. One such patient characteristic appears to be the phoria status; it appears that bifocal control of myopia is more likely in children with esophoria at near. Studies on the effect of bifocals on childhood myopia progression are summarized in Tables 6.1 and 6.2. In the one study on the effect of bifocals on young adulthood myopia progression, Shotwell (1981, 1984) did not find a statistically significant reduction in myopia progression rates in military academy students with bifocals.

Studies Analyzing Private Practice Patient Records

Mandell (1959) selected records of 175 myopic patients from an optometry practice in California who had two or more refractions before age 30 years. The mean initial ages of the patients were 14.3 years in those wearing bifocals and 17.1 years in those who had not worn bifocals; therefore, many of the patients in Mandell's analysis would have already had a completion of their childhood myopia progression. On the basis of visual inspection of large composite x,y plots of myopia as a function of age, Mandell concluded that bifocals did not prevent further progression of myopia. These graphs are published in the paper and show that Mandell's conclusion is justified. However, visual inspection of plots for numerous subjects on one graph is not as precise as the calculation of rates of myopia progression in determining whether there may be some reduction in rates of myopia progression with bifocals as opposed to a complete stoppage.

Miles (1962) often prescribed 28-mm flat-top segment bifocals for myopia patients in his ophthalmology practice in St. Louis. He also generally decentered the lenses to give a small base-in prism effect. Data were presented for 103 patients who wore single vision lenses and 48 patients who wore bifocal lenses after an initial period of single vision lens wear. Miles states that the mean rate of myopia progression before the use of bifocals was approximately –0.75 D per year for age spans of 6–14 years. These patients then progressed at a rate of –0.40 D per year over age spans of 8–16 years when wearing bifocals. Part of the difference in rates with and without bifocals could be accounted for by the difference in ages. However, inspection of the graphs published by Miles of mean myopia as a function of age suggests that myopia was progressing more slowly with bifocals over common age spans.

Roberts and Banford (1963, 1967) selected data for myopic patients refracted at least twice before the age of 17 years from the files of their three optometry practices in New York State. They obtained records of 47 girls and 38 boys who wore bifocal lenses exclusively over the observation period. Patients wearing single vision lenses numbered 231 females and 165 males. The powers of the plus additions in the bifocals varied between +0.75 and +2.00 D, with most of them being +1.50 D adds or less. Roberts and Banford calculated myopia progression rates in diopters per year based on the mean of the spherical equivalent manifest subjective refractions in the two eyes. They found that the mean rates of progression decreased as a

TABLE 6.1
Summary of Studies on the Use of Bifocals for Myopia Control in Children

Study	Number, Ages, and Location of Subjects	Type and Power of Bifocal	Rates of Progression in D/yr with SV	Rates of Progression in D/yr with BF	Summary of Results and Interpretation
Miles (1962)	SV: n = 103, ages 6–14 yrs; SV then BF: n = 48, ages 8–16 years; St. Louis	28-mm wide flat-top segments, decentered for slight base-in effect	-0.75	-0.40	Inspection of graphs suggests lower rates with BF over common age spans
Oakley and Young (1975)	SV: n = 298; BF: n = 269; Members of both groups ages 6–17 yrs at start of study; Oregon	Flat-top segments with top at pupil center; +1.50 to +2.00 D adds	Whites: -0.53 Native Americans: -0.38	Whites: -0.02 Native Americans: -0.10	Largest reported reduction of rate with BF of all studies
Neetens and Evens (1985)	SV: n = 733; BF: n = 543; Patients who had myopia of <0.50 D at 8 or 9 years of age; Holland	For myopia up to 3 D: total near point power equal to zero; For myopia 3 D or more: +2.50 D add	-0.45	-0.30	Mean amount of myopia at age 18 yrs was less for BF wearers (-3.55 D) than for SV wearers (-5.07 D)
Schwartz (1976, 1981)	25 monozygotic twin pairs, one of each in BF and one in SV group; age 7–13 yrs at start of study; Washington, DC	+1.25 D add	-0.27	-0.24	Difference in rates for SV and BF groups not statistically significant; overall rate lower than rates found in other studies

TABLE 6.1
Continued

Study	Number, Ages, and Location of Subjects	Type and Power of Bifocal	Rates of Progression in D/yr with SV	Rates of Progression in D/yr with BF	Summary of Results and Interpretation
Grosvenor et al. (1987)	SV: $n = 39$ BF (+1.00 D add): $n = 41$ BF (+2.00 D add): $n = 44$ Members of all groups ages 6–15 yrs at start of study Houston	Executive bifocals*; top of reading segment 2 mm below pupil center	–0.34	+1.00 D adds: –0.36 +2.00 D adds: –0.34	Mean rate not significantly different in either BF group from SV group
Pärssinen et al. (1989)	SV full-time wear: $n = 79$ SV distance use: $n = 79$ BF: $n = 79$ Mean beginning age: 10.9 yrs in each group Finland	28-mm-wide segments with +1.75 D add; top of segment 2–3 mm below pupil center	–0.57 (mean of both eyes, both SV groups)	–0.53 (mean of both eyes)	Mean rate not significantly different in BF group from either SV group
Jensen (1991)	SV: $n = 49$ BF: $n = 51$ Children in second through fifth grades at start of study Denmark	35-mm-wide segment with +2.00 D add; top of segment at lower pupil margin	All: –0.57 IOP ≤16: –0.43 IOP ≥17: –0.66	All: –0.48 IOP ≤16: –0.47 IOP ≥17: –0.49	For children with IOP ≥17 mm Hg, rates were less with BF than with SV

SV = single vision lenses; BF = bifocal lenses; IOP = intraocular pressure.
* American Optical Co., Southbridge, MA.
Source: Modified from DA Goss. Effect of spectacle correction on the progression of myopia in children. J Am Optom Assoc 1994;65:117–128.

TABLE 6.2
Summary of Studies on the Use of Bifocals for Myopia Control in Children—Studies in which von Graefe Near Phorias Were Measured

Study	Number, Ages, and Location of Subjects	Type and Power of Bifocal	Rates of Progression in D/yr with SV	Rates of Progression in D/yr with BF
Roberts and Banford (1963, 1967)	SV: n = 396; BF: n = 85; Members of both groups examined at least twice before age 17 yrs; New York State	Most adds were +0.75 to +1.50 D	All: -0.41; Ortho and exo: -0.41; Eso: -0.48	All: -0.31; Ortho and exo: -0.38; Eso: -0.28
Goss (1986)	SV: n = 52; BF: n = 60; Age 6–15 yrs; Illinois, Iowa, Oklahoma	Most adds were +0.75 and +1.00 D	Ortho and exo: -0.44; Eso: -0.54	Ortho and exo: -0.45; Eso: -0.32
Goss and Grosvenor (1990)	SV: n = 32; BF: n = 65; Age 6–15 yrs; Reanalysis of Grosvenor et al. data from Houston	Executive bifocals*; +1.00 and +2.00 D adds	Ortho and exo: -0.44; Eso: -0.51	Ortho and exo: -0.42; Eso: -0.31
Fulk and Cyert (1996)	SV: n = 14; BF: n = 14; Boys: age 6.00–13.99 yrs; Girls: age 6.00–12.99 years at start of study; all had esophoria at near; Oklahoma	28-mm-wide flat-top segments; +1.25 D adds; top of segment 1 mm above lower limbus	Eso: -0.57	Eso: -0.39

SV = single vision lenses; BF = bifocal lenses.
*American Optical Co., Southbridge, MA.
Source: Modified from DA Goss. Effect of spectacle correction on the progression of myopia in children. J Am Optom Assoc 1994;65:117–128.

function of age. Such a finding is to be expected, because children with earlier ages of myopia onset have higher rates of progression, and mean rates after the mid-teens would be reduced due to some of the patients' having a cessation of their childhood myopia progression. Therefore, to eliminate age as a variable, they adjusted rates using a formula derived from correlation analysis for the relationship of age and rate. The mean rates of progression were –0.31 D per year for the bifocal wearers and –0.41 D per year for the single vision lens wearers. The difference in means was statistically significant at the 0.02 level.

Oakley and Young (1975) presented data for myopic patients from Oakley's ophthalmology practice in central Oregon, which served white and American Indian patients. Oakley routinely recommended bifocal lenses to all children with myopia. In the Oakley and Young data, the control group consisted of children who wore single vision lenses because either they or their parents had refused bifocals. The distance portion of the bifocals, as well as the single vision lenses, typically contained a 0.50 D undercorrection of the patient's myopia. The near addition in the bifocals was usually a +1.50 to +2.00 D flat-top segment with the top of the segment at pupil center with the eyes in primary position. Bifocal and single vision lens wearers were matched by age and amount of myopia in the paper. Mean rates of progression for the right eye of white patients were –0.02 D per year among the 226 bifocal wearers and –0.53 D per year in the 215 who used single vision lenses. The mean rates in American Indian patients were –0.10 D per year for 43 in bifocals and –0.38 D per year for 83 wearing single vision lenses.

The amount of reduction in progression rates with bifocals was greater in the Oakley and Young study than in any other report, which they attributed to the high placement of the reading portion of the lens in the spectacle frame. Another potential partial explanation is a high prevalence of esophoria in their sample. Oakley and Young stated that "virtually all children fitted with bifocals in this study demonstrated a nearpoint esophoria, as did most of the control children who were progressing," although such a great preponderance of esophoria does seem unusual. Oakley and Young also noted that inadvertent examiner bias may have affected study results.

Neetens and Evens (1985) reported data for myopic children whom they examined between 1959 and 1982 in the University of Antwerp Department of Ophthalmology in Holland. The report included children who initially had myopia of 1.00 D or less at age 8 or 9 years. Exclusion criteria were astigmatism (amount of astigmatism not stated), anisometropia of more than 1 D, and moderate or large amounts of exophoria or esophoria. The test distance and method of measurement for phoria testing were not stated. The bifocal near add power that they prescribed varied with the amount of myopia. The total nearpoint power was plano for patients with myopia of less than 3 D. Patients with 3.0 D of myopia or greater were given bifocals with near additions of +2.50 D. The mean manifest subjective refraction at age 18 years for both eyes of 733 single vision lens wearers was –5.07 D (range, –4.50 to –10.50 D). The mean refractive error at age 18 years for 543 bifocal wearers was –3.55 D (range, –3.00 to –8.50 D). Ninety-seven percent of the single vision lens group had refractions in the range of –4.50 to –6.50 D at 18 years, whereas 97% of the bifocal group were in the range of –3.00 to –5.00 D. Neetens and Evens stated that the amount of myopia at age 18 years in the single vision lens group and the bifocal group were significantly different by the Yates and Cochran statistical test ($p < .001$). If we assume that the amount of myopia at the beginning was 0.50 D, the rates of myopia progression would have been approximately –0.45 D per year for the single vision lens group and –0.30 D per year for the bifocal group.

Prospective Studies Conducted in Clinics

Monozygotic twins served as subjects in a study by Schwartz (1976, 1981). Twelve female twin pairs and 13 male twin pairs completed the 3½-year study. One member of each twin pair was in the experimental group and the other was in the control group. The treatment for the experimental group consisted of wearing bifocal spectacle lenses with +1.25 D near additions and instilling one drop of 1% tropicamide in each eye at bedtime. Due to the short duration of action of tropicamide, it seems unlikely that there was any significant cycloplegic or mydriatic effect during the waking hours. The inclusion criteria for the subjects were age 7–13 years, bilateral myopia, 20/20 or better corrected visual acuity, third-degree fusion, 1.00 D or less astigmatism, 1.00 D or less anisometropia, no other significant ocular anomaly, good general health, and a difference in refractive error from the other member of the twin pair of no more than 1.50 D in the more myopic eye. Average binocular mean cycloplegic spherical equivalent refractions at the beginning of the study were –2.33 D in the bifocal group and –2.22 D in the single vision lens group. The mean myopia progression for all 50 subjects was –0.26 D per year. Schwartz stated that the difference in rates for the two study groups was 13% of the rate for all the subjects, making the difference approximately 0.03 D per year less in the bifocal group, which was not statistically significant. For the 15 twin pairs with higher rates of progression, the reduction in rate with bifocals was 16% of the rate for all these subjects with higher rates, a difference that was not statistically significant. The rates of myopia progression were much lower in this study than in other childhood myopia progression studies.

In a study conducted at the University of Houston College of Optometry (Grosvenor et al., 1985, 1987; Young et al., 1985), subjects were randomized to one of three groups: a single vision lens control group, a +1.00 D add bifocal group, and a +2.00 D add bifocal group. The bifocal lenses were CR-39 plastic Executive bifocals with the top of the reading segment 2 mm below the center of the subject's pupil. The power of the distance portion of the bifocal lenses was equal to the binocular maximum plus subjective refraction to best visual acuity. That was also the power of the single vision lenses, which were made of polycarbonate material. Eligibility criteria at the beginning of the study were 6–15 years of age, spherical equivalent refractive error of at least 0.25 D of myopia, normal visual acuity, normal binocular vision, normal ocular health, and no contact lens wear. One hundred twenty-four (58 males and 66 females) of the 207 subjects who started the study completed its full 3-year duration. The rates of myopia progression based on the difference in the first and last right eye spherical equivalent refractions divided by three were single vision lens group (n = 39), –0.34 D per year; +1.00 D add bifocal group (n = 41), –0.36 D per year; and +2.00 D add bifocal group (n = 44), –0.34 D per year.

An ophthalmology group in Finland (Hemminki and Pärssinen, 1987; Pärssinen and Hemminki, 1988; Pärssinen et al., 1989) enrolled study subjects based on the following criteria: spherical equivalent refractive error in the range of –0.25 to –3.00 D, anisometropia not greater than 2.00 D, astigmatism not greater than 2.00 D, no strabismus, Maddox wing horizontal phorias between 10Δ exo and 9Δ eso, vertical phoria not more than 1Δ, no previous spectacle lens wear, no ocular disease, and no serious systemic disease. The treatment groups were (1) full-time wear of single vision lenses containing power equal to a full correction of the subject's myopia, (2) distance vision use of single vision lenses containing a full correction, and (3) bifocals with a +1.75 D add in a 28-mm wide flat-top reading segment. The top of the reading segment was placed 2–3 mm below pupil center. Each of the three groups had mean subject ages of 10.9 years at the beginning of the study. At the end of the study, 79 subjects remained in each study group, with follow-up times that varied from 2.0 to 5.1 years. The follow-up periods were 3.0–3.1 years for 95% of the subjects. The refractive data used for analysis were subjective refractions done 45–60 minutes after the instillation of two drops of 1% cyclopentolate. Mean right eye changes in spherical equivalent refractive error were –1.48 D (SD = 0.9) in the full-time wear single vision lens group, –1.76 D (SD = 1.0) in the distance-wear single vision lens group, and –1.67 D (SD = 0.9) in the bifocal group. Mean left eye changes were –1.46 D (SD = 0.9) in the group that wore single vision lenses full-time, –1.88 D (SD = 1.0) in the group that wore single vision lenses for distance vision, and –1.58 D (SD = 0.9) in the group that used bifocal lenses. The differences in mean changes between the bifocal group and the full-time single vision lens group were not statistically significant.

A Danish ophthalmologist (Jensen, 1991) attempted myopia control with two forms of treatment with children who were in second through fifth grades and had myopia of –1.25 to –6.00 D at the start of the study. Subjects in the control group wore single vision lenses. One treatment group consisted of children who wore plastic bifocal lenses with a +2.00 D power near lens addition in a 35-mm wide reading segment. The top of the bifocal segment was positioned at the lower pupil margin with the eyes in straightforward position. The other treatment was single vision lens wear and daily administration of timolol eye drops. Right eye spherical equivalent Topcon autorefractor readings after instillation of 1% cyclopentolate were the refractive data used for statistical analysis. The mean amounts of change in myopia in 2 years were –1.14 D (*n* = 49, SD = 0.71) in the control group, –0.95 D (*n* = 51, SD = 0.56) in the bifocal group, and –1.18 D (*n* = 45, SD = 0.59) in the timolol group. Mean changes in the two treatment groups did not differ significantly from the mean change in the control group.

An interesting finding from Jensen's (1991) study was that myopia progression was less with bifocals than with single vision lenses in children who had intraocular pressures of 17 mm Hg or above at the beginning of the study. The mean refractive changes for subjects with the higher intraocular pressure readings were –1.32 D (*n* = 27, SD = 0.70) in the control group, –0.97 D (*n* = 24, SD = 0.64) in the bifocal group, and –1.19 D (*n* = 23, SD = 0.58) in the timolol group. Intraocular pressure was lowered in the timolol group, but mean myopia progression in the timolol group did not differ significantly from that in the control group.

The studies discussed so far have found variable success, some showing myopia control with bifocals and some not. Among the many possible explanations for the variable study results could be differences in add powers, segment heights, study populations, inclusion criteria, compliance to the use of the reading portion of the lenses, or other factors. Another potential explanation is that bifocals may give more effective myopia control in some types of cases than in others. As discussed next, there is evidence that bifocals slow myopia progression in children with nearpoint esophoria, but not in children with exophoria at near.

Effect of Phoria Status on Reduction of Progression Rates with Bifocals

Miles (1962) graphed the mean amount of myopia as a function of age for groups of patients separated by Maddox rod distance phoria. Estimates of the slopes of the graphs for the 6- to 15-year age span (Goss, 1994) for patients who wore single vision lenses over the whole time span were –0.35 D per year in 18 exophores, –0.27 D per year for 31 orthophores, and –0.51 D per year for 54 esophores. Miles fit children with higher rates of myopia progression with bifocals. Eighteen patients with orthophoria or exophoria had progression rates of –0.77 D per year before use of bifocals and –0.51 D per year with bifocals. Thirty patients with distance esophoria had progression rates of –0.73 D per year before bifocals were used and –0.38 D per year after bifocal wear began.

Roberts and Banford (1963, 1967) found less myopia progression with bifocals than with single vision lenses in children with nearpoint esophoria on the von Graefe dissociated phoria test. Mean myopia progression rates in esophoria were –0.48 D per year (*n* = 167) for single vision lens wearers and –0.28 D per year (*n* = 65) for bifocal lens wearers. Rates in orthophoria and exophoria were –0.41 D per year (*n* = 181) with single vision lenses and –0.38 D per year (*n* = 17) with bifocals. Myopia control with bifocals was also greater in higher accommodative convergence–to–accommodation (AC/A) ratio cases. AC/A ratios were calculated using the distance and near von Graefe phorias. Patients with AC/A ratios of less than 5.0 Δ/D had mean rates of –0.44 D per year (n = 84) in the single vision lens group and –0.41 D per year in the bifocal wearers. Mean rates for patients with AC/A ratios of 9.0 Δ/D or greater were –0.59 D per year (n = 39) with single vision lenses and –0.31 D per year (n = 19) with bifocal lenses; in other words, 0.28 D per year lower with bifocals. In cases with AC/A ratios from 5.0 to 6.9 Δ/D, rates were only 0.08 D per year less with bifocals, and with AC/A ratios of 7.0–8.9 Δ/D, rates were 0.12 D lower with bifocals.

Goss (1986) collected patient data from three optometry practices in the central United States. Records were selected based on the following criteria: at least four refractions between the ages of 6 and 15 years, myopia of at least 0.50 D, astigmatism of 2.50 D or less, no strabismus or amblyopia, no contact lens wear, no ocular disease, and no systemic disease that might affect ocular findings. Rates of myopia progression in diopters per year were calculated by linear regression using points from ages 6 to 15 years. Refractive error data used for analysis were the lens powers in the right eye principal meridian nearest horizontal from the manifest subjective refraction. Phoria data were obtained by the von Graefe test through the manifest subjective refraction lenses. The mean rates of progression for patients with nearpoint orthophoria or exophoria were –0.44 D per year (n = 36) in single vision lens wearers and –0.45 D per year (n = 21) in bifocal lens wearers. When patients with esophoria at near were considered, rates were significantly (p <.05) lower in bifocal wearers (mean = –0.32 D per year; n = 35; SD = 0.20) than in single vision lens wearers (mean = –0.54 D per year; n = 10; SD = 0.30).

The data from the University of Houston study were reanalyzed by Goss and Grosvenor (1990). This reanalysis differed from the initial data analysis (Grosvenor et al., 1987) in that only examinations between ages 6 and 15 years were used, rates were calculated by linear regression, and mixed astigmats were not included. When subjects with orthophoria or exophoria were considered, the mean progression rates were –0.44 D per year (n = 25) for single vision lens wearers and –0.42 D per year (n = 47) for bifocal lens wearers. Mean rates were –0.51 D per year (n = 7; SD = 0.22) for esophores wearing single vision lenses and –0.31 D per year (n = 18; SD = 0.31) for esophores wearing bifocal lenses. The difference in rates between the single vision group and the bifocal group for esophoric subjects was not statistically significant due to the small sample size, but the magnitude of the difference was the same as the 0.20 D per year difference found by Roberts and Banford (1963, 1967) and very similar to the 0.22 D per year difference found by Goss (1986).

Jensen (1991), who used the cover test with a 30-cm test target to determine near phoria, did not find the same magnitude of difference between bifocal-wearing esophores and single vision lens–wearing esophores as did Roberts and Banford (1963, 1967), Goss (1986), and Goss and Grosvenor (1990). The latter three studies all used the von Graefe test with a 40-cm test target. Similar results to the latter three studies were found by Fulk and Cyert (1996), who also used the von Graefe test to determine phoria status.

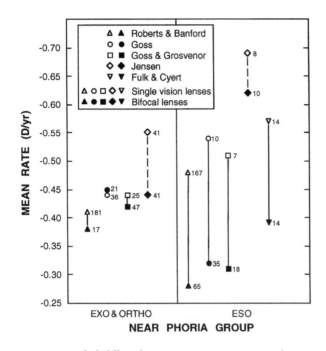

FIGURE 6.1. Mean rates of childhood myopia progression as a function of spectacle lens type and near phoria, from five studies. Rates with single vision lenses are represented by open symbols; rates with bifocals are represented by filled symbols. The numbers by each point represent the numbers of patients. In the Jensen study (points connected by dashed lines), phoria status was determined by cover test with a 30-cm test distance. In the other studies (points connected by solid lines), phorias were measured with the von Graefe test with a near point card test target at 40 cm.

In the Fulk and Cyert study (1996), myopic subjects used either single vision lenses or bifocal lenses with a +1.25 D add in a 28-mm wide flat-top segment. Subjects were followed for 18 months. One of the subject inclusion criteria was esophoria at near on the von Graefe test. Refractive data used for analysis were the mean of the spherical equivalents of the two eyes from autorefraction after the instillation of two drops of 1% tropicamide. The mean rates of myopia progression were –0.57 D per year (n = 14; SE = 0.11) for the single vision lens group and –0.39 D per year (n = 14; SE = 0.12) for the bifocal group. The difference between groups was not statistically significant due to the small sample size. The magnitude of the difference (0.18 D per year) was very similar to that found by the previously named studies, as shown in Figure 6.1.

Goss and Uyesugi (1995) expanded the database used for an earlier study (Goss, 1986) by adding data from three additional practices. Data analysis methods were the same as in the previous study. The mean rates for children with orthophoria or exophoria at near were –0.42 D per year

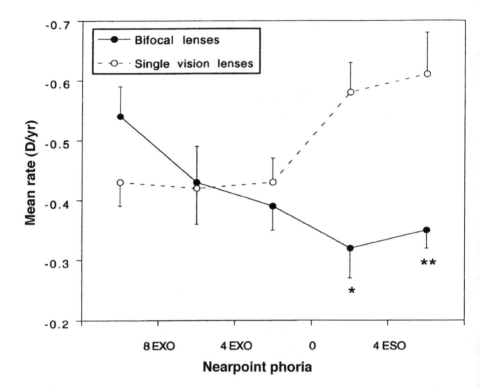

FIGURE 6.2. Mean rates of childhood myopia progression as a function of spectacle lens type and near phoria, from Goss and Uyesugi (1995). Error bars are one standard error. Asterisks indicate that the means for the bifocal group and the single vision lens group were significantly different by t-test (*p <.001; **p <.0005). (Reprinted with permission from DA Goss, EF Uyesugi. Effectiveness of bifocal control of childhood myopia progression as a function of near point phoria and binocular cross-cylinder. J Optom Vis Dev 1995;26:12–17.)

(n = 103) for single vision lens wearers and –0.44 D per year (n = 55) for bifocal lens wearers. Considering patients with nearpoint esophoria, mean rates were –0.59 D per year (n = 52; SD = 0.32) for the single vision lens group and –0.33 D per year (n = 66; SD = 0.20) for the bifocal group. The mean rate for the bifocal group was significantly less than that for the patients who used single vision lenses (p <.000002). Rates as a function of near phoria from this study are illustrated in Figure 6.2.

The studies in which phorias were measured with the von Graefe technique are summarized in Table 6.2. The mean rates of myopia progression were approximately 0.20 D per year less with bifocals when the near phoria was eso. There was no difference in rates between the two lens types when the near phoria was either ortho or exo.

☼ CLINICAL PEARL

In four studies, bifocal lenses reduced the mean rate of childhood myopia progression by approximately 0.20 D per year in patients with esophoria at near. This was a reduction in rate of approximately 40%, and over a period of 5 years would result in approximately 1 D less myopia.

Progressive Addition Lenses

Studies are now under way that examine the effect of progressive addition lenses on childhood myopia progression, but to date there appears to have been only one study completed. Man (1997) followed 68 children at Hong Kong Polytechnic University for 2 years. Thirty-two subjects wore single vision lenses; 22 subjects wore progressive addition lenses with +1.50 D reading adds; and 14 used progressive addition lenses with +2.00 D adds. The mean myopia progression in 2 years in the single vision lens group was –1.23 D (SD = 0.51). The mean progression in 2 years in the +1.50 D add group was –0.76 D per year (SD = 0.43), and in the +2.00 D add group, it was –0.66 D per year (SD = 0.44). The amounts of progression were significantly less in both the +1.50 D add group (p <.001) and the +2.00 D add group (p <.0005) than in the single vision lens group.

Undercorrection

A study in Japan (Tokoro and Kabe, 1964, 1965) compared myopia progression rates in children wearing full corrections of their myopia to that in children wearing undercorrections of more than 1 D. The mean rate for full correction was –0.75 D per year (n = 13; SD = 0.27), and for undercorrection it was –0.54 D per year (n = 10; SD = 0.39). The difference was statistically significant. One potentially confounding factor in this study was that some subjects in each group were also receiving pharmaceutical treatments for attempted myopia control. When only subjects who were not receiving other treatments were considered, the mean rates were 0.83 D per year (n = 11; SD = 0.18) with full correction and –0.47 D per year (n = 5; SD = 0.09) with undercorrection. These means were also significantly different, although with such low numbers of subjects, unknown selection factors may have affected the results. Undercorrections of more than 1 D, as used in this study, would, of course, reduce the clarity of distance vision.

Part-Time Wear of Spectacles

The study by Pärssinen et al. (1989), discussed earlier, included a treatment group in which subjects wore a full correction of their myopia for distance vision use only. The rates of progression for that group (given earlier) do not show a myopia control effect.

Tokoro and Kabe's study (1965) also included a group of subjects who wore their full correction part time. The mean rates of progression were –0.75 D per year (*n* = 13; SD = 0.27) in the full-time full-correction group and –0.62 D per year (*n* = 10; SD = 0.32) in the part-time full-correction group. These means were not significantly different, but the fact that several of the subjects also received other treatments makes the results difficult to interpret.

Summary of Study Results

Although the results of studies on the efficacy of bifocals for myopia control have been variable, one consistent finding so far is an average reduction in myopia progression rates of approximately 0.2 D per year in children with esophoria at near on the von Graefe test. Bifocals do not appear to control myopia in children with orthophoria or exophoria at near. The use of plus adds for near in nearpoint esophoria can be justified not only for myopia control, but also for providing more comfortable binocular vision (Birnbaum, 1993; Scheiman and Wick, 1994; Goss, 1995).

One study reported significant myopia control with progressive addition lenses. One study did not find myopia control to occur with use of full correction for distance vision only. The data on undercorrection as a potential method of myopia control are very limited.

Power to Use in Bifocals

The previous studies do not give an obvious answer as to the power that is most beneficial for myopia control. Earlier, it is discussed that two studies found that rates of childhood myopia progression were lowest for patients with near phorias in the normal range of approximately ortho to 6Δ exo. On that basis, it may be advisable for patients with eso at near to prescribe an add that would bring their near phoria into the normal range. Because most of the variability in near phoria is related to variability in AC/A ratio, the adds used will not be highly variable; most often an add of +1.00 to +1.50 would be needed to shift a near eso into the ortho to low exo range.

Comments on Patient Education

Patients and parents of young children know that bifocals and progressive addition lenses ("no-line bifocals") are used for patients with presbyopia (older persons), but they may not be aware that such lenses are often used for nonpresbyopes (persons of their own age or younger). In presenting bifocal lens wear to nonpresbyopes or to parents, it is best to first present the concept of the patient benefiting from different lens powers for distance and near, rather than using the word *bifocal* initially. A demonstration is often very helpful because patients with convergence excess, esophoria at near, and/or accommodative insufficiency will almost always see print more clearly and comfortably with a plus add than with their distance correction. It can be demonstrated by the practitioner that one lens power is better for distance and the other is better for near. It can then be mentioned to the patient, parents, or both that the way that different lens powers can be achieved in one lens is with a bifocal or a progressive addition lens.

☀ **CLINICAL PEARL**

A theoretically sound approach to prescribing near adds for myopia control in children with nearpoint esophoria is to prescribe just enough plus to shift the near phoria into the ortho to low exo range. Usually, this can also be demonstrated to the patient as providing clearer and/or more comfortable near vision.

References

Birnbaum MH. Optometric Management of Nearpoint Vision Disorders. Boston: Butterworth–Heinemann, 1993.

Fulk GW, Cyert LA. Can bifocals slow myopia progression? J Am Optom Assoc 1996;67:749–754.

Goss DA. Effect of bifocal lenses on the rate of childhood myopia progression. Am J Optom Physiol Opt 1986;63:135–141.

Goss DA. Effect of spectacle correction on the progression of myopia in children—a literature review. J Am Optom Assoc 1994;65:117–128.

Goss DA. Ocular Accommodation, Convergence, and Fixation Disparity: A Manual of Clinical Analysis (2nd ed). Boston: Butterworth–Heinemann, 1995.

Goss DA, Grosvenor T. Rates of childhood myopia progression with bifocals as a function of near point phoria: consistency of three studies. Optom Vis Sci 1990;67:637–640.

Goss DA, Uyesugi EF. Effectiveness of bifocal control of childhood myopia progression as a function of near point phoria and binocular cross-cylinder. J Optom Vis Dev 1995;26:12–17.

Grosvenor T, Maslovitz B, Perrigin DM, Perrigin J. The Houston myopia control study: a preliminary report by the patient care team. J Am Optom Assoc 1985;56:636–643.

Grosvenor TP, Perrigin DM, Perrigin J, Maslovitz B. Houston myopia control study: a randomized clinical trial. Part II. Final report by the patient care team. Am J Optom Physiol Opt 1987;64:482–498.

Hemminki E, Pärssinen O. Prevention of myopia progress by glasses. Study design and the first year results of a randomized trial among schoolchildren. Am J Optom Physiol Opt 1987;64:611–616.

Jensen H. Myopia progression in young school children. A prospective study of myopia progression and the effect of a trial with bifocal lenses and beta blocker drops. Acta Ophthalmol 1991;(Suppl 200):1–79.

Man JLT. The effect of progressive lenses on the progression of myopia in Chinese school children. M.Ph. Thesis, The Hong Kong Polytechnic University, 1997.

Mandell RB. Myopia control with bifocal correction. Am J Optom Arch Am Acad Optom 1959;36:652–658.

Miles PW. A study of heterophoria and myopia in children, some of whom wore bifocal lenses. Am J Ophthalmol 1962;54:111–114.

Neetens A, Evens P. The use of bifocals as an alternative in the management of low grade myopia. Bull Soc Belge Ophtalmol 1985;214:79–85.

Oakley KH, Young FA. Bifocal control of myopia. Am J Optom Physiol Opt 1975; 52:758–764.

Pärssinen O, Hemminki E. Spectacle use, bifocals, and prevention of myopic progression—the two years' results of a randomized trial among schoolchildren. Acta Ophthalmol 1988;66(Suppl 185):156–161.

Pärssinen O, Hemminki E, Klemetti A. Effect of spectacle use and accommodation on myopic progression: final results of a three-year randomized clinical trial among schoolchildren. Br J Ophthalmol 1989;73:547–551.

Roberts WL, Banford RD. Evaluation of Bifocal Correction Technique in Juvenile Myopia. OD dissertation. Massachusetts College of Optometry, 1963.

Roberts WL, Banford RD. Evaluation of Bifocal Correction Technique in Juvenile myopia. Optom Weekly 1967;58(38):25–28,31; 58(39):21–30; 58(40):23–28; 58(41):27–34; 58(43):19–24,26.

Scheiman M, Wick B. Clinical Management of Binocular Vision: Heterophoria, Accommodative, and Eye Movement Disorders. Philadelphia: Lippincott, 1994.

Schwartz JT. A monozygotic cotwin control study of a treatment for myopia. Acta Genet Med Gemellol 1976;25:133–136.

Schwartz JT. Results of a Monozygotic Cotwin Control Study on a Treatment for Myopia. In L Gedda, P Parisi, WE Nance (eds), Twin Research 3: Epidemiological and Clinical Studies. New York: Liss, 1981;249–258.

Shotwell AJ. Plus lenses, prisms, and bifocal effects on myopia progression in military students. Am J Optom Physiol Opt 1981;58:349–354.

Shotwell AJ. Plus lenses, prism, and bifocal effects on myopia progression in military students, Part II. Am J Optom Physiol Opt 1984;61:112–117.

Tokoro T, Kabe S. Treatment of the myopia and the changes in optical components. Report I. Topical application of Neosynephrine and tropicamide. Acta Soc Ophthalmol Jpn 1964;68:1958–1961.

Tokoro T, Kabe S. Treatment of the myopia and the changes in optical components. Report II. Full- or under-correction of myopia by glasses. Acta Soc Ophthalmol Jpn 1965;69:140–144.

Young FA, Leary GA, Grosvenor T, et al. Houston myopia control study: a randomized clinical trial. Part I. Background and design of the study. Am J Optom Physiol Opt 1985;62:605–613.

CHAPTER 7

Myopia Control with Pharmaceutical Agents

No discussion of myopia control or reduction would be complete without mentioning attempts to control the progression of myopia by means of various pharmaceutical agents. Unfortunately, the evidence that cycloplegic agents, sympathetic blocking agents, or other pharmaceuticals have a significant effect in reducing the progression of myopia without unwanted side effects is not at all convincing. The results of clinical studies—especially those using atropine to control progression in children—have shown that the agent would have to be instilled daily for the 5- to 10-year period during which myopia would be expected to progress.

Cycloplegic Agents

Because many practitioners and vision scientists believe that myopia is caused by accommodation during near work, the literature contains a number of studies making use of cycloplegic agents for myopia control. Many problems can arise during long-term use of cycloplegic agents. These include the following:

1. The inconvenience of instilling drops on a daily basis for a period of several years
2. The necessity to remove glasses for reading or to wear bifocals or reading glasses
3. Constant photophobia due to pupillary dilation, unless photochromic or other absorptive lenses are worn
4. The high possibility of an adverse reaction to the cycloplegic agent or of interaction with systemic medication
5. The ethical problem of prescribing long-term medication for a child who is in good health

In addition to these well-known adverse effects, it is possible that atropine may be toxic to retinal cells. Crewther et al. (1985) reported that chronic atropinization of kittens led to reduced resolving power of the ganglion cells.

Atropine

The authors of most of the clinical studies of atropine for myopia control—including Curtin (1970), Gimbel (1973), Bedrossian (1979), and Gruber (1979)—did not mention the use of bifocals or reading glasses. However, Bedrossian's subjects instilled atropine in just one eye, so the other eye could be used for near work. In the last two atropine studies described here—those of Sampson (1979) and Brodstein et al. (1984)—bifocals were used along with the atropine drops.

In a pilot study reported by Curtin (1970), 10 myopic children instilled one drop of 1% atropine in one eye every evening for 6 months, with the other eye as a control. At the end of the 6-month period, the children were kept under observation for an additional 6 months. At the end of the one-year period, the difference in progression rates for treated and control eyes was only 0.05 D.

In the first large-scale study to be reported, Gimbel (1973) compared the progression of myopia for 279 experimental subjects and 572 controls. The mean ages of the experimental and control subjects were 9.7 and 11.0 years, respectively. The usual dosage was one drop of 1% atropine in each eye at night, but this was sometimes reduced if reading difficulties were reported, and was reduced or increased depending on whether the myopia had stabilized or was progressing. Gimbel's report is confusing, contradictory, and difficult to interpret. He stated that 53% of the patients had stopped treatment, usually because of "annoying side effects," but he also stated that only 22 of the original 279 treated subjects were followed for 3 years. Furthermore, Gimbel reported results for only those treated subjects who initially presented with myopia no greater than –2.00 D, and for control subjects whose initial myopia was no greater than –1.50 D. For the 22 treated subjects, the mean change in refractive error was 0.07 D less myopia, whereas for the control subjects (number not reported), there was a mean increase in myopia of 1.22 D. Interpretation is further complicated by the fact that refractive error was measured under atropine cycloplegia for the treated subjects but under tropicamide cycloplegia for the control subjects.

Gruber (1979) reported results of a study involving a treatment group of 100 myopic children who received one drop of 1% atropine daily, and a control group of 100 myopic children. The dropout rate was reported to be 12%. The treatment group progressed at a mean rate of 0.11 D per year during a treatment period of 1–2 years, and at a mean rate of 0.46 D per year after treatment. The control group progressed at a mean rate of 0.28 D per year. Thus, for the treated subjects the mean progression rate during the 2-year period was $0.5 \times (0.11 + 0.46)$, or 0.29 D, per year. This is similar to the progression rates in the absence of treatment, indicating that the retarded rate of progression during atropine treatment was compensated by the accelerated rate of progression once treatment had ceased.

Bedrossian (1979) used a crossover study design in which subjects instilled 1% atropine into one eye for a 1-year period, and in the fellow eye during the following year. Refraction was measured under atropine cyclo-plegia for the treated eye but under tropicamide cycloplegia for the control eye. For 90 subjects who remained in the study for 2 years, the mean change in refractive error was 0.20 D less myopia for the treated eyes and 0.94 D more myopia for the control eyes. For the two eyes of each subject, this indicates a mean rate of myopic progression of $0.5 \times (-0.20 + 0.94)$, or 0.37 D, per year. For the 28 subjects who remained in the study for an additional 2 years, the mean changes in refractive error were 0.30 D less myopia for the treated eyes and 0.90 D more myopia for the control eyes, indicating a mean progression rate of $0.5 \times (-0.30 + 0.90)$, or 0.30 D, per year. For the 57 subjects who were examined between 1 and 6 years after completion of the study, the mean progression rate was 0.06 D per year.

The value of atropine treatment in the Bedrossian (1979) study is questionable because the mean progression rates of 0.37 D per year for the first 2 years and 0.30 D per year for the third and fourth years of the study differed little from the expected progression rate for children of comparable ages in the absence of any treatment. For example, in the Grosvenor et al. (1987) bifocal study, members of the single vision lens–wearing control group progressed at a mean rate of 0.34 D per year. Moreover, Bedrossian's mean post-treatment progression rate of 0.06 D per year, which occurred when the subjects were between 12 and 22 years of age, is consistent with the finding that myopic progression generally stops or slows down during the middle teen years (Goss and Winkler, 1983).

Studies Using Atropine and Bifocals

In a study in which 112 myopic children served as treatment subjects but with no control group, Sampson (1979) used one drop of 1% atropine daily in combination with bifocals. For periods of up to 12 months, he reported that for 79% of subjects the refractive error changed between –0.25 and +0.50 D. For periods of 6–12 months after discontinuation of treatment, myopia was found to progress at a rapid rate (more than 1.00 D in some cases). Sampson concluded that atropine does not stop the progression of myopia, but only delays it.

The effect of combining atropine and bifocals for myopia control was examined by Brodstein et al. (1984). The treatment group consisted of 435 myopic children who were fitted with +2.25 D add bifocals and given one drop of 1% atropine in each eye every morning; the control group consisted of 146 myopic children who wore single vision lenses and did not receive atropine. The follow-up period averaged 33 months for the treated subjects and 49 months for the control subjects. The treatment group progressed at a mean rate of 0.16 D per year during the treatment period and 0.38 D per year after treatment, for a mean progression rate of 0.23 D per year. The control group progressed at a mean rate of 0.25 D per year. Again, this study failed to demonstrate that atropine reduces the rate of myopic progression.

Tropicamide

Abraham (1966) compared progression rates for 68 myopic children age 7–18 years who instilled 1% tropicamide drops at bedtime, and a control group of 82 myopic children. The two groups were matched for age, sex, and family history of myopia. Abraham's rationale was that the use of the eyes for near work during the daytime resulted in a "spastic ciliary muscle" during the night, and the advantage of instilling tropicamide drops at bedtime was that the children were not likely to be bothered by pupillary dilation or poor accommodation during the daytime. Bifocals were not used, but the children were encouraged to read without their glasses if necessary. Abraham commented that the children's pupils were seldom still dilated on rising in the morning, and if near work was required early in the morning, "the uncorrected nearsightedness took care of the problem." Over an 18-month observation period, the mean progression rates were 0.27 D per year for the experimental group and 0.57 D per year for the control group. Although this is a reduction rate of approximately 50%, Jensen and Goldschmidt (1991) suggested that it is difficult to draw any conclusions from this study because all untreated children, regardless of reason, were placed in the control group.

Schwartz (1976, 1981) described an 8.5-year study involving the use of both tropicamide and bifocals. Subjects for the study were 25 pairs of myopic monozygotic twins between 7 and 13 years of age. One twin in each pair wore bifocals with a +1.25 D add and was given two drops of 1% tropicamide in each eye at night, while the other twin wore single vision lenses and did not receive tropicamide. Schwartz reported that the mean rate of progression for all subjects was 0.26 D per year and that the mean progression rate was 0.03 D per year less for the treatment group than for the control group. This small difference is obviously not clinically significant. The extended duration of the study and the use of identical twins are positive aspects of the design of this study. Although no treatment effect appears to have occurred, the overall low rate of progression may have made a treatment effect less likely to be observed.

The results of studies using cycloplegic agents for myopia control are summarized in Table 7.1.

TABLE 7.1
Summary of the Results of Studies Using Cycloplegic Agents for Myopia Control

Study	Subjects	Duration	Mean Change in Refraction		
			Treatment	Control	Post-Treatment
Atropine					
Curtin (1966)	10[a]	6 mos	See below[b]	—	Not reported
Gimbel (1973)	22 T[b]	3 yrs	None	–0.41 D/yr	Not reported
Gruber (1979)	100 T 100 C	1–2 yrs (variable)	–0.11 D/yr	–0.28 D/yr	–0.46 D/yr
Bedrossian (1979)	90[c] 28	2 yrs 4 yrs	+0.10 D/yr +0.15	–0.47 D/yr –0.45 D/yr	–0.06 D/yr[d]
Sampson (1979)	112 T 0 C	12 mos	See below[e]	—	See below[e]
Brodstein et al. (1984)	435 T 146 C	Mean of 3 yrs Mean of 7 yrs	–0.16 D/yr	–0.25 D/yr	–0.30 D/yr
Tropicamide					
Abraham (1966)	68 T 82 C	18 mos	–0.27 D/yr	–0.57 D/yr	Not reported
Schwartz (1975, 1981)	25 T[f] 25 C	8.5 yrs	–0.24 D/yr	–0.27 D/yr	Not reported

C = control; T = treatment.
[a]Fellow eye used as control. Mean difference in change in refractive error was 0.05 D.
[b]Number of controls completing the study not given. Data reported only for experimental subjects with initial refraction of no greater than –2.00 D and controls with initial refraction of no greater than –1.50 D.
[c]Crossover study; fellow eye used as control (in alternate years).
[d]The 57 post-treatment subjects were examined after 1–6 years, at ages 12–22 years.
[e]Seventy-nine percent of subjects changed from –0.25 to +0.50 D but progressed rapidly after discontinuation of treatment.
[f]Subjects were monozygotic twins: One of each pair of twins was in the treatment group and the other was in the control group.

⚞ **CLINICAL PEARL**

In view of the difficulties resulting from the regular instillation of the cycloplegic drugs already described—that is, inconvenience, reading problems, photophobia, the possibility of adverse reactions to the drug, and the ethical problems associated with the instillation of a potentially harmful substance into a healthy eye— as well as the lack of convincing evidence that either atropine or tropicamide is effective in myopia control or reduction, there appears to be no reason to engage in this form of therapy.

Adrenergic Blocking Agents

The rationale for the use of adrenergic blocking agents for myopia control is based on the supposition that axial elongation and myopia are due to increased intraocular pressure (IOP) and that by reducing the IOP these agents should reduce the rate of myopia progression.

Adrenergic blocking agents that have been used for this purpose include labetalol, a beta-adrenergic antagonist that also exhibits weak alpha-adrenergic blocking action, and the nonspecific beta-antagonist timolol maleate. Hosaka (1988) reported results of a study of 50 myopic children ages 6–14 years who were given 0.5% and 0.25% labetalol twice daily; 16 children acted as controls. After 2–4 months of treatment, the refractive error for the treated subjects decreased by a mean of 0.40 D, and there was apparently no change in refractive error for the control subjects. In the same article, Hosaka (1988) reported that 0.25% timolol drops were given twice daily to 20 myopic children ages 7–14 years of age, with 16 children acting as controls. After 2–6 months of treatment, there was no significant effect on myopia progression, with only 28% of patients having a reduction in myopia of at least 0.25 D. Post-treatment data were not reported in either of these short-term studies.

In a 2-year prospective clinical trial reported by Jensen (1991), 159 children ages 9–12 years were randomly assigned to a timolol group, a bifocal group, and a single vision control group. At the end of the 2-year period, 145 children remained in the study, 49 of whom were in the control group, 51 in the bifocal group, and 45 in the timolol group. The difference in mean progression rates for the timolol group (0.59 D per year) and the single vision control group (0.57 D per year) was not statistically significant, although a decrease in mean IOP was found in the timolol group. Timolol instillation was discontinued after 2 years, and at the end of an additional year, both the timolol and control groups were found to progress at a mean rate of 0.42 D per year.

The results of studies making use of adrenergic blocking agents for myopia control are summarized in Table 7.2.

☼ CLINICAL PEARL
There is no convincing evidence that adrenergic blocking agents are effective in myopia control or reduction.

Future Possibilities: Agents Acting on the Retina

It has been shown that some pharmaceutical agents may act at the retinal level in addition to (or instead of) the ciliary muscle level. Atropine, pirenzepine, and apomorphine, all of which have been found to act on the retinas of some species, have been used for the purpose of blocking the development of experimentally induced myopia.

TABLE 7.2
Summary of the Results of Studies Using Adrenergic Blocking Agents
for Myopia Control

			Mean Change in Refraction		
Study	*Subjects*	*Duration*	*Treatment*	*Control*	*Post-Treatment*
Labetalol					
Hosaka	50 T	2–4 mos	+0.40 D	Not	Not
(1988)	16 C			reported	reported
Timolol					
Hosaka	20 T	2–6 mos	See below[a]	Not	Not
(1988)	16 C			reported	reported
Jensen	145[b]	2 yrs	–0.59 D/yr	–0.57 D/yr[c]	–0.42 D/yr
(1991)					

C = control; T = treatment.
[a]No significant effect.
[b]The 145 subjects who completed the study had been randomized into a timolol group, a bifocal group, and a single vision control group.
[c]For the single vision control group.

Atropine

Whereas newly hatched chicks that are monocularly deprived by means of a translucent occluder are found to develop myopia, McBrien et al. (1993) found that intravitreal injection of atropine blocked the development of myopia. They concluded that because chick intraocular muscles are striated and contain mainly nicotinic as opposed to muscarinic receptors, atropine may block myopia in chicks via a nonaccommodative (i.e., retinal) mechanism. McBrien et al. suggested that any effect of atropine in blocking myopia in humans might also be due to a retinal mechanism.

Pirenzepine

Leech et al. (1995) reported that experimental myopia in chicks monocularly deprived by the use of hemispherical plastic occluders can be inhibited by intravitreal or subconjunctival injection of pirenzepine, which is an M1 muscarinic antagonist that acts on the chick retina.

Apomorphine

To determine if retinal dopamine could be relevant to ocular development in chicks, Stone et al. (1989) locally administered apomorphine, a dopamine antagonist, to lid-sutured chicks and found that it inhibited axial elongation in a dose-dependent manner. Iuvone et al. (1988) topically applied apomorphine in lid-sutured rhesus monkeys and found that it retarded axial elongation and the development of myopia. They concluded that "the apparent activity of apomorphine drops in a primate species suggests that its use, or the use of related dopamine receptor agonists, might be a therapeutic strategy for study in modifying the development of certain human myopias."

As of this writing, there have been no reports of the use of retinally active agents for the control or reduction of human myopia.

References

Abraham SV. Control of myopia with tropicamide. A progress report. Ophthalmology 1996;3:10–22.

Bedrossian, RH. The effect of atropine on myopia. Ophthalmology 1979;86:713–717.

Brodstein RS, Brodstein DE, Olson RJ, et al. The treatment of myopia with atropine and bifocals. Ophthalmology 1984;91:1373–1379.

Crewther DP, Crewther SG, Cleland BG. Is the retina sensitive to the effects of prolonged blur? Exp Brain Res 1985;58:427–434.

Curtin BJ. Myopia: a review of its etiology, pathogenesis and treatment. Surv Ophthalmol 1970;15:1–17.

Gimbel HV. The control of myopia with atropine. Can J Ophthalmol 1973;8:527–532.

Goss DA, Winkler RL. Progression of myopia in youth: age of cessation. Am J Optom Physiol Opt 1983;60:651–658.

Grosvenor T, Perrigin DM, Perrigin J, Maslovitz B. Houston myopia control study: a randomized clinical trial. Part 2. Final report of the patient care team. Am J Optom Physiol Opt 1987;64:482–498.

Gruber E. The Treatment of Myopia with Atropine: A Clinical Study. In ET Shimizu, JA Oosterhuis (eds), Ophthalmology, Proceedings of the XXIII International Congress. Kyoto, May 14–20, 1978. Amersterdam: Excerpta Medica, 1979; 1212–1216.

Hosaka A. The role of pharmaceutical agents. Acta Ophthalmologica 1988;185 (Suppl 66):130–131.

Iuvone PM, Tigges M, Stone RA, et al. Effects of apomorphine, a dopamine receptor agonist, on ocular refraction and axial elongation. Invest Ophthalmol Vis Sci 1988;31:1674–1677.

Jensen H. Myopia progression in young school children. A prospective study of myopia progression and the effect of a trial with bifocal lenses and beta blocker eye drops. Acta Ophthalmol 1991;(Suppl 200):1–79.

Jensen H, Goldschmidt E. Management of Myopia: Pharmaceutical Agents. In T Grosvenor, M Flom (eds), Refractive Anomalies: Research and Clinical Applications. Boston: Butterworth–Heinemann, 1991;371–383.

Leech EM, Cottraill CL, McBrien NA. Pirenzepine prevents form deprivation myopia in a dose dependent manner. Ophthalmic Physiol Opt 1995;15:351–356.

McBrien NA, Moghaddam HO, Reeder AP. Atropine reduces experimental myopia and eye enlargement via a nonaccommodative mechanism. Invest Ophthalmol Vis Sci 1993;34:205–215.

Sampson WG. Role of cycloplegia in the management of functional myopia. Ophthalmol 1979;86:695–697.

Schwartz JT. A monozygotic cotwin control study of a treatment for myopia. Acta Genet Med Gemellol 1976;25:133–136.

Schwartz JT. Results of a Monozygotic Cotwin Control Study on a Treatment for Myopia. In L Gedda, P Parisi, WE Nance (eds), Twin Research 3: Epidemiological and Clinical Studies. New York: Liss, 1981;249–258.

Stone RA, Lin T, Laites AM, Iuvone PM. Retinal dopamine and form-deprivation myopia. Proc Nat Acad Sci USA 1989;86:704–706.

CHAPTER 8

Corneal Topography Measurement

Information concerning corneal topography is useful in routine contact lens fitting and is especially valuable in orthokeratology and in the management of keratorefractive surgery patients. A keratometer of the Bausch & Lomb (B&L; Rochester, NY) design measures a portion of the cornea having a chord diameter of approximately 3 mm. Beyond this 3-mm zone, the cornea is known to gradually flatten toward the periphery, usually measuring approximately 0.6–1.0 mm (3.00–5.00 D) flatter in the periphery than at the apex. Methods that may be used to investigate the topography of the cornea include peripheral keratometry, photokeratoscopy, and videokeratoscopy.

Peripheral Keratometry

The simplest method of using the keratometer to obtain information concerning the corneal topography is to use the "plus" and "minus" signs on the B&L keratometer mire as fixation points. The central keratometer reading is first taken in the usual manner, and the patient is then asked to fixate, in turn, the two plus signs (to the left and right) and the two minus signs (above and below). With each new fixation, the keratometer is realigned so that the crosshairs are in the center of the undeviated mire image. For the fixation points to the left and right, only the reading in the principal meridian nearest 180 degrees is recorded; for the upper and lower fixation points, only the reading in the principal meridian nearest 90 degrees is recorded. Although the readings taken in this manner are not quantitatively accurate (as discussed below), they are helpful in giving the practitioner information concerning *relative amounts of peripheral flattening* in each semimeridian of the cornea. The advantage of using the plus and minus signs as fixation points is that they measure areas of the cornea

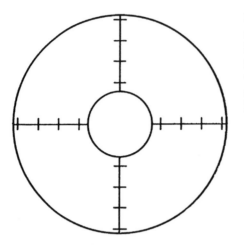

FIGURE 8.1. A plastic "K-disk" designed to fit on the front of a Bausch & Lomb keratometer, providing fixation points for peripheral keratometry. (Reprinted with permission from T Grosvenor. Contact Lens Theory and Practice. Chicago: Professional Press, 1961;19.)

that are approximately *4.5 mm from the corneal apex*, which is about as far in the periphery as measurements are possible on most corneas—even with the expensive videokeratoscopes.

To obtain more complete information concerning the corneal topography, auxiliary fixation points may be provided by the use of a simple plastic "K-disk." Such a disk, shown in Figure 8.1, has four fixation points in each semimeridian, located 14, 21, 28, and 35 mm from the center of the keratometer mire plate and corresponding to points on the corneal surface approximately 2, 3, 4, and 5 mm from the corneal apex. After taking the central keratometer reading in the usual manner, the examiner instructs the patient to sequentially fixate each of the four fixation points to the left, to the right, upward, and downward, realigning the instrument for each change in fixation. For fixation points to the left and right, only the reading in the principal meridian closest to 180 degrees is recorded; for fixation points upward and downward, only the reading in the principal meridian closest to 90 degrees is recorded.

Once the readings have been taken and recorded, they are plotted on a graph as shown in Figure 8.2, which can be done by the use of a computer graphics program. The graph enables the examiner to estimate the position of the corneal apex, the width of the optic zone (the zone in which there is no more than 1 D of flattening as compared with the central keratometer reading), and the amount of the peripheral flattening in the cornea's principal meridians. For example, the data plotted in Figure 8.2 (taken from a report by Grosvenor [1961]) indicate a well-centered corneal apex; an optic zone that is approximately 2 mm wide horizontally and 4 mm wide vertically; and peripheral flattening of approximately 3.00 D nasally and temporally, 3.50 D in the lower cornea, and 2.50 D in the upper cornea.

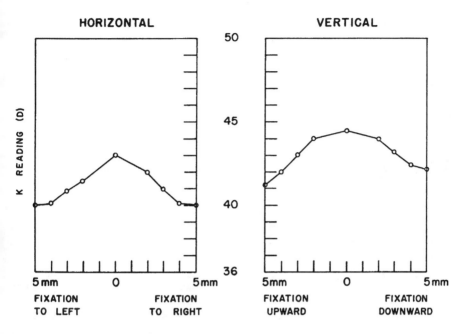

FIGURE 8.2. A typical graph of peripheral keratometry data. With such a graph, the position of the corneal apex, the width of the optic zone, and the amount of peripheral flattening can be estimated. (Reprinted with permission from T Grosvenor. Contact Lens Theory and Practice. Chicago: Professional Press, 1963;19.)

Peripheral Keratometry in Contact Lens Practice

Data taken by means of a K-disk can sometimes be very useful in the fitting of rigid contact lenses. Whereas the topography of the cornea of a typical contact lens candidate would be very much like that shown in Figure 8.2, one occasionally encounters a cornea that has a misplaced apex or has little or no peripheral flattening. For example, in the report referred to above (Grosvenor, 1961), a prospective contact lens wearer's cornea was found to have no peripheral flattening and an upward-displaced apex, as shown in Figure 8.3. We found that it was impossible to fit this eye with the "standard" polymethyl methacrylate (PMMA) contact lens, having an overall diameter of approximately 9.5 mm and a secondary curve approximately 1 mm flatter than the base curve (which allows for the expected peripheral flattening of the cornea). On the basis of the topographic data, a decision was made to fit a lens that was virtually all optic zone (parallel to the central keratometer reading) with only a narrow edge-bevel. A satisfactory fit was obtained with this lens.

Although peripheral keratometry data can often be very useful in the fitting of rigid contact lenses, it should be understood that there are some

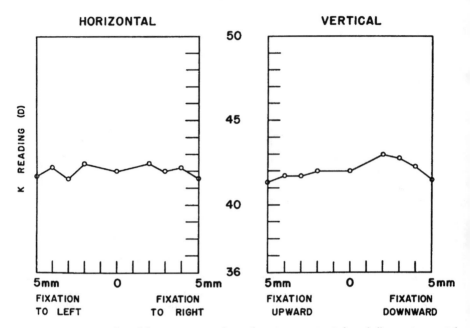

FIGURE 8.3. Peripheral keratometry data showing no peripheral flattening, with the corneal apex displaced upward. (Reprinted with permission from T Grosvenor. Contact Lens Theory and Practice. Chicago: Professional Press, 1963;27.)

inherent sources of error. Because the keratometer does not measure the curvature (and hence the refracting power) at a specific point on the cornea, but measures the curvature between two points that are approximately 3 mm apart, when we are measuring the curvature in the midperiphery of the cornea, one measuring point (plus or minus sign) may be very close to the corneal apex and the other may be relatively far in the periphery. A second source of error is that the computations used in designing peripheral keratometry targets assume that the center of rotation of the eye is a fixed point with respect to the eye, whereas it actually varies with the position of the eye. A third source of error is that the centers of curvature of the various peripheral areas of the cornea are not located along the optic axis of the cornea.

In spite of these inherent errors, peripheral keratometry can be of value in fitting rigid contact lenses on corneas having unusual topographies. There is no reason to use peripheral keratometry on all corneas before fitting contact lenses. However, peripheral keratometry readings should be considered whenever routine methods, such as fluorescein pattern interpretation, fail to result in a successful fit. As discussed below, photokeratoscopy and videokeratoscopy are alternative, although much more expensive, methods of obtaining information concerning corneal topography prior to contact lens fitting.

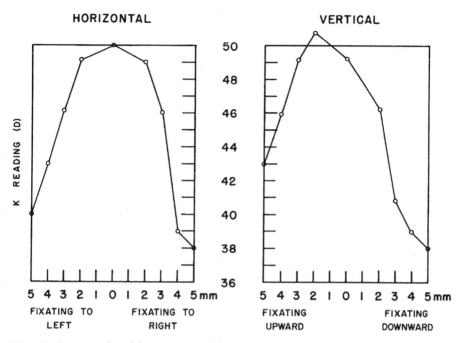

FIGURE 8.4. Peripheral keratometry data for an eye with keratoconus. The corneal apex is displaced 2–3 mm downward, with a very large amount of peripheral flattening. (Reprinted with permission from T Grosvenor. Contact Lens Theory and Practice. Chicago: Professional Press, 1963;330.)

☼ **CLINICAL PEARL**
The fluorescein pattern will normally serve as a guide in obtaining a successful rigid lens fit, but there are cases in which this is not true. If the desired fluorescein pattern and/or optimal centration and blink lag are not obtained, the cause of the problem and its solution can almost always be found by performing peripheral keratometry.

Detection of Keratoconus

Some insight into corneal topography in keratoconus can be gained from Figure 8.4 (Grosvenor, 1963), which shows a corneal apex that is decentered downward approximately 1 mm, an optic zone no larger than 2 mm, and peripheral flattening of 10–12 D nasally and temporally and 7–12 D in the lower and upper cornea. Such an eye requires a lens with a very small optic zone and a series of increasingly flatter secondary and peripheral curves. Although neither photokeratoscopy nor videokeratoscopy was available when this patient was examined, it is doubtful that either of these procedures would have provided additional information of any importance.

Photokeratoscopy

Instrumentation designed specifically for measurement of the corneal topography had its beginnings in 1880 with *Placido's disk*, which forms an image of a concentric-ring target on the cornea. Placido's disk does not allow for quantification of corneal toricity or peripheral flattening: in fact, the reflected rings, as viewed by the examiner, appear to be perfectly circular for an eye having as much as 2 D of corneal astigmatism. In 1924, Gullstrand developed the first photokeratoscope by mounting a Placido's disk target on the base of an instrument that looks very much like a keratometer, and attaching a camera. Using this instrument, Gullstrand concluded that the normal cornea had an optical zone width of approximately 4 mm, decentered slightly downward and outward and that the peripheral cornea flattened nasally more than temporally and upward more than downward.

Reynolds (1959) developed what he called a *Photo-Electronic keratoscope* (Wesley Jessen, Des Plaines, IL). This instrument used high magnification to measure the concentric ring photographs, and this information was used to determine the specifications (optic zone size, peripheral curve radii and width) for the patients' contact lenses. A later version of the photokeratoscope, called the *Cornea-Scope* (Kera Corporation, Santa Clara, CA), was developed during the 1970s. As described by Rowsey et al. (1981), this instrument produces a Polaroid photograph, from which the dioptric power at the corneal apex and at various peripheral points is read by the use of a comparator that magnifies the picture 4.1–6.3 times to match it to a standard set of rings on the comparator screen. The CorneaScope was widely used in ophthalmic practice before the introduction of computerized videokeratoscopes. For example, it was used to analyze the changes in corneal topography as a result of radial keratotomy (RK) surgery, in the prospective evaluation of RK study (Rowsey et al., 1988).

Videokeratoscopy

Klyce and his colleagues developed a system of digitizing keratoscope photographs and using the data to reconstruct the three-dimensional shape of the cornea; this required 5,000–8,000 data points, from which the radius of curvature was calculated for selected points (Klyce, 1984; Maguire et al., 1987). From these radius values, the keratometric index of refraction of 1.3375 was used to calculate dioptric values. Using this information, a color-coded contour map of the distribution of corneal power was plotted. In these maps, cool colors indicate low corneal powers, whereas warm colors indicate higher corneal powers. The usual range of colors, from low to high corneal powers, is from violet to blue to green to yellow to orange to red. In the original instrument, the "step-size"—that is, the dioptric change from one color to the next—could be a minimum of 1.5 D, whereas for later instruments smaller step-sizes became available.

TABLE 8.1
Videokeratoscopy Instruments

Instrument	Manufacturer	Location
Eye Map EH 290	Alcon Surgical	Ft. Worth, TX
Keratron Corneal Analyzer	Alliance Medical Marketing	Jacksonville Beach, FL
CT-200	Dicon	San Diego, CA
ET-800	Euclid Systems Corp.	Herndon, VA
Corneal Analysis System	EyeSys Technologies	Houston, TX
Atlas 990	Humphrey Instruments	San Leandro, CA
Orbscan	Orbtek	Salt Lake City, UT
CTS and Acu-Grid	PAR Vision Systems	New Hartford, NY
KR-7000P	Topcon America Corp.	Paramus, NJ

Source: Modified from 20th Annual Instruments Report: corneal topographers. Rev Optom 1997;134:95–96.

The original Klyce instrument was marketed by Computed Anatomy, Inc., New York, as the *Corneal Modeling System*, but this instrument was replaced in the early 1990s by the *Topographical Modeling System*. In recent years, many other instruments have become available. Currently available videokeratoscopy instruments are listed in Table 8.1.

The Corneal Modeling System was used in a study by Bogan et al. (1990) that was designed to classify the topography of the normal cornea. Topographic measurements were made on 409 normal eyes of 217 subjects. In an analysis of the color-coded topographic maps, five qualitatively different patterns were found. Black-and-white reproductions of examples of these patterns are shown in Figure 8.5. A *round pattern* was found in 23% of eyes, an *oval pattern* in 21%, a *symmetric bow-tie pattern* in 17%, an *asymmetric bow-tie pattern* in 32%, and an *irregular pattern* in 7% of eyes. The only variables that showed statistically significant differences among the patterns were keratometric and refractive astigmatism. As one might expect, the round and oval patterns were associated with relatively spherical corneas, whereas the bow-tie (both symmetric and asymmetric) was associated with keratometric astigmatism. The irregular pattern did not show a statistically significant difference in keratometric astigmatism from the other patterns except the symmetric bow-tie pattern. Bogan et al. concluded that "[c]lassification of normal corneal topography is an important step in the process of characterizing the shape of normal and pathologic corneas."

Accuracy of Topographic Maps

In spite of the fact that the cornea is subject to spherical aberration, Roberts (1994) reported that dioptric power maps produced by videokerato-

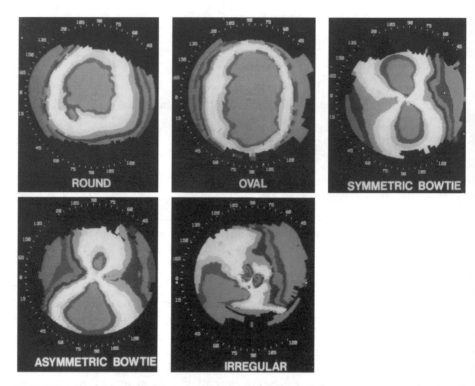

FIGURE 8.5. Black-and-white reproduction of topographic map patterns. (Reprinted with permission from SJ Bogan, GO Waring, O Ibraham, et al. Classification of normal corneal topography based on computer assisted videokeratography. Arch Ophthalmol 1990;108:945–949.)

scopic data are inappropriately based on *paraxial equations*. On the basis of ray-tracing, Roberts has shown that, whereas paraxial corneal power is the reciprocal of the secondary focal length, paraxial corneal power may be approximated by either of two methods. The first approximation, called *axial power*, is given by $(n - 1)/d$, where n is 1.3375 and d is the *axial radius*, the distance from the corneal surface to the corneal axis. The second approximation, called *instantaneous power*, is given by $(n - 1)/r$, where r is the *instantaneous* radius, the distance from the corneal surface to the center of curvature of the surface. Because of peripheral flattening, the instantaneous radius is longer than the axial radius. However, for a spherical surface, $d = r$, and both the first and second approximations are equal to the actual refracting power. According to Roberts, the instantaneous power formula was originally used by Klyce for topographic devices, but it has since been shown that these devices do not accurately measure the instantaneous radius of curvature, more closely modeling the axial radius.

On the basis of calculations for corneas having eccentricity values of 0.3 and 0.5 (recall that a circle has an eccentricity of zero, and a parabola has an eccentricity of 1.0), Roberts stated that "[t]he surprising results of this study indicate that not only is the error significant, the paraxial power approximations actually produce a completely opposite pattern from the corneal refracting power. In both ellipsoids, where the paraxial approximations show decreasing values, the corneal refracting power is actually increasing!" She suggested that manufacturers of instrumentation for videokeratoscopy should label their color-coded maps in terms of curvature (presumably, the reciprocal of the radius of curvature) rather than refracting power.

Salmon and Horner (1995) have extended the work of Roberts by applying it to toric corneas. Suggesting that the color-coded maps resulting from videokeratoscopy data should be called *dioptric curvature* maps rather than power maps, they designed a theoretical "model cornea" having a constant shape factor (equal to $1 - e^2$, where e is eccentricity) of 0.85, and apical radii of 8.00 mm horizontally and 7.50 mm vertically, resulting in 2.81 D of with-the-rule astigmatism. For each corneal point, sagittal depth was calculated. On the basis of this information, they produced color-coded maps for axial curvature, instantaneous curvature, and raytrace refracting power. These results demonstrated, again, that due to the cornea's spherical aberration, refracting power *increases* toward the periphery in spite of the fact that curvature *decreases* toward the periphery.

Salmon and Horner suggested that a simple solution to the problem of interpreting the color-maps would be to discontinue using the paraxial formula and to leave the radii in millimeters, but "since clinicians are not likely to abandon diopters as a descriptor for corneal topography, we recommend that axial and instantaneous dioptric data be interpreted as curvature, rather than power."

Comparison of Videokeratoscopy and Peripheral Keratometry

At Indiana University, Buege et al. (1996) obtained both central and peripheral corneal data on 20 eyes of 19 subjects, using the Marco (B&L design) keratometer and the EyeSys Corneal Analysis System (EyeSys Technologies, Houston, TX). The subject population was made up of 10 normal eyes with no history of contact lens wear; seven eyes of current wearers of daily wear soft contact lenses; one eye of a former soft contact lens wearer; and both eyes of a former PMMA lens wearer who had recently been diagnosed as having keratoconus. Except for the keratoconic subject, data were taken on only one eye of each subject. With the keratometer, the central reading was first taken in the usual manner, with the subject fixating the red fixation light. After this, peripheral keratometer readings were taken with the aid of a plastic K-disk, using the procedure described earlier in this chapter. EyeSys data were then taken, using the procedure described by the manufacturer of the instrument.

Both the keratometer and the EyeSys data were plotted on graphs similar to those shown for peripheral keratometry data in Figure 8.2. For the

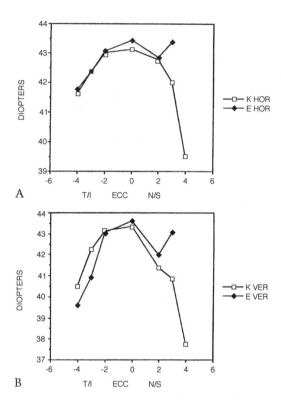

FIGURE 8.6. Comparison of peripheral keratometry data and EyeSys data for a typical eye. (A) Horizontal meridian. (B) Vertical meridian. (T/I = temporal or inferior cornea; ECC = eccentricity; N/S = nasal or superior cornea; open symbols = keratometer; closed symbols = Eye-Sys; K HOR = keratometer horizontal meridian; E HOR = EyeSys horizontal meridian; K VER = keratometer vertical meridian; E VER = EyeSys vertical meridian.) (Reprinted with permission from T Buege, R Hanna, T Grosvenor. Comparison of corneal topography obtained by keratometry and videokeratoscopy. Int Contact Lens Clin 1996;23:142–148.)

keratometer, the data were plotted by means of a Cricket Graphics program, using a Macintosh computer, whereas for the EyeSys, the data were plotted by means of the EyeSys program. For many of the 20 eyes, the plots for the data generated by the keratometer and the EyeSys were remarkably similar, more so in the horizontal meridian than the vertical meridian. Data for a typical eye are shown in Figure 8.6. For some eyes, the EyeSys data showed localized irregularities that were not shown in the keratometer data. Possible reasons for such "blips" could be the presence of a corneal irregularity caused by mucous or other debris in the tear film, or (in vertical meridian data) by the superior or inferior marginal tear strip. For example, the steeper EyeSys data point shown in Figure 8.6B (3 mm above the corneal apex) may have been due to the superior marginal tear strip. As for the subject who had recently been diagnosed as having bilateral keratoconus, the graphs for the keratometer data and the EyeSys data were very similar, indicating (for both eyes) that the "cone" was decentered downward 2 mm.

Because the data resulting from the keratometer and the EyeSys were so similar, Buege et al. (1996) concluded that when videokeratoscopy is not available, peripheral keratometry can provide useful information concerning the corneal topography.

Applications of Videokeratoscopy

Videokeratoscopy can be useful in many ophthalmic procedures, including rigid contact lens fitting, orthokeratology, and keratorefractive surgery.

Applications in Rigid Contact Lens Fitting

In an editorial titled "Computerized videokeratography: just pretty pictures or a valuable clinical tool?" Lowther (1994) raised a question that must be in the minds of many practitioners. He asked whether instruments for this purpose, costing from $20,000 to $35,000, have sufficient clinical value to justify their purchase by the typical practitioner.

Among the points made by Lowther included the following:

1. There are mechanical problems in actually capturing the image, including poor focusing and misalignment, which can cause significant errors.
2. The representation of the corneal contour is particularly helpful with keratoconus patients, corneal distortion problems, fitting contact lenses after refractive surgery, and other related problems.
3. If used for designing the fit of a rigid contact lens, the instruments in conjunction with their software do not result in accurate fits in a high percentage of patients.
4. One limitation is that the software does not take into account lid positions and other dynamics.
5. Corneal topographers have not replaced fluorescein pattern evaluation and professional judgment, although they may aid the astute fitter.

The last two points made by Lowther—that the instruments and their software do not always result in accurate fits and that the programs do not take lid position and other dynamics into consideration—are particularly important. For the astute practitioner, the fluorescein pattern not only provides information concerning the fit of the lens (too flat, too steep, too large, too small, etc.), but provides crucial information concerning lens position and blink lag.

Lester et al. (1994) compared the results of videokeratoscope and conventional rigid gas-permeable (RGP) lens fitting and found that the failures with the videokeratoscope method were due to a combination of base curves that were too flat, optic zone diameters that were too small, secondary curves that were too flat, and peripheral curves that were too flat. They concluded that because of high cost and limited success, current videokeratoscope software systems for contact lens design are of limited value, although they can be of great benefit in RGP problem solving.

Maeda and Klyce (1994) suggested a number of situations in which videokeratoscopy can be useful in the fitting of contact lenses. These include the detection of irregular astigmatism (which may occur as a result of keratoplasty, trauma or advanced keratoconus), detection of contact lens–induced corneal warpage, screening refractive surgery candidates for keratoconus, creating computer simulations of fluorescein patterns, and assessing the optical quality of worn soft contact lenses. However, before the advent of videokeratoscopy, all these situations could be easily cared for by keratometry (including the simplified form of peripheral keratometry in which readings are taken while the patient fixates the "plus and minus signs" on the keratometer mire); therefore, in our opinion, there is no reason for a practitioner to purchase a videokeratoscope unless he or she wishes to monitor refractive surgery patients.

☼ CLINICAL PEARL

Videokeratoscopy has little to offer in the realm of RGP contact lens fitting. Computer programs designed for this purpose are less likely to achieve a successful fit than the careful application of time-honored procedures, including the use of the keratometer, fluorescein pattern interpretation, and the evaluation of lens position and lag.

Applications in Conventional Orthokeratology

In conventional orthokeratology, in which conventional rigid contact lenses are sequentially fitted increasingly flatter in order to flatten the optic zone of the cornea, the end stage of the procedure occurs when the corneal periphery is no longer flatter than the optic zone—that is, when "sphericalization" of the cornea has occurred. Ordinary keratometry is the method of choice for monitoring the flattening of the optic zone, and simplified peripheral keratometry is an appropriate method for determining when sphericalization has taken place.

Applications in Accelerated Orthokeratology
Using "Reverse Geometry" Lenses

As described in Chapter 9, the aim of this form of orthokeratology is to flatten the optic zone of the cornea while simultaneously steepening the midperiphery. Depending on the practitioner's preference, these curvature changes can be monitored either by a combination of central and peripheral keratometry or by videokeratoscopy. If a practitioner emphasizes accelerated orthokeratology, comanagement of refractive surgery in his or her practice, or both, the purchase of a videokeratoscope may prove to be a good investment.

Applications in Keratorefractive Surgery

The question of whether videokeratoscopy is necessary for the performance of keratorefractive surgery was addressed at a symposium organized by the New Orleans Academy of Ophthalmology. As reported by Maguire (1994), there was general agreement among participants that videokeratoscopy provides the surgeon with so much information that cannot be obtained by a keratometer or other instrumentation, that there is no point in trying to get along without it. In the case of RK and excimer laser photorefractive keratectomy (PRK) (see Chapter 10), videokeratoscopy is used as a part of the presurgical screening procedure and for postsurgical monitoring. Therefore, if an optometrist wishes to comanage keratorefractive surgery patients, access to videokeratoscopy is a must.

Preoperative Screening for Keratoconus

Maeda and Klyce (1994) urged that videokeratoscopy should be used to screen keratorefractive surgery patients for keratoconus, inasmuch as RGP contact lenses—rather than refractive surgery—are indicated for keratoconic eyes. Although the prevalence of keratoconus is not high, it is likely that keratoconus patients are overrepresented in the population of candidates for keratorefractive surgery: This population includes a high proportion of contact lens wearers who are unsatisfied with their contact lens fit or with the resulting vision, or both. For example, it was reported by Nesburn et al. (1992) that in a study of 91 patients presenting for refractive surgery, 7% had a pattern of corneal topography consistent with early keratoconus.

Moreover, it is likely that the prevalence of keratoconus is much higher than was formerly thought. The problem of screening for keratoconus before undertaking refractive surgery has been discussed by Maguire (1994). He introduced his discussion with the question, "Who would want to perform refractive surgery on a cornea that has the potential to develop severe instability or distortion even without surgery?" He answered the question by saying that this is exactly what will happen if a patient with subclinical keratoconus is operated on. Maguire cited studies showing that rather than being a very rare condition that occurs sporadically, keratoconus is a much more prevalent autosomal dominant condition. For example, Rabinowitz et al. (1990) reported that 50% of nonsymptomatic family members of keratoconic patients showed topographic findings that were consistent with early keratoconus.

Maguire (1994) also addressed the issue of what the refractive surgeon should look for when using videokeratoscopy for the screening of early keratoconus. He referred to a report by Wilson et al. (1991), who found two major topography patterns in keratoconus: Approximately 75% of keratoconic eyes showed a peripheral cone, which was most commonly located in an inferior quadrant, while approximately 25% showed a central cone.

Screening for Changes in Corneal Topography Due to Contact Lens Wear

Because a high percentage of candidates for keratorefractive surgery are contact lens wearers, it is imperative that the practitioner screen refractive surgery candidates for disturbances in the corneal topography due to contact lens wear. Both rigid and soft contact lenses are known to cause such disturbances. Rigid lenses sometimes cause a long-term corneal flattening, along with corneal "warpage," which often induces as much as 2 or 3 D of with-the-rule corneal astigmatism. In some cases, this is *irregular* astigmatism, in which the two principal meridians are not orthogonal. The induced astigmatism is almost always present centrally and can easily be found by routine keratometry; however, if the patient's refractive history is not available, it may be uncertain whether the astigmatism was induced by the contact lenses or was present before the lenses were fitted. In any case, videokeratography will provide useful information. In discussing rigid contact lens–induced corneal warpage, Maguire (1994) noted that corneal mapping of eyes of patients with symptomatic corneal warpage showed changes that were indistinguishable from those of early peripheral keratoconus.

Experience has shown that corneal distortion due to rigid lenses can persist for as long as 3–6 weeks after the cessation of contact lens wear. Most rigid lens wearers who have severe corneal distortion are those who do not have a wearable pair of glasses and therefore wear their contact lenses during all of their waking hours. The best way to deal with such a situation is to have the patient reduce his or her wearing time—over a period of a week or two—to approximately 8 hours per day. At this time, the corneas will have stabilized sufficiently so that glasses can be prescribed and wearing time can then be reduced to zero over a period of another week or two. At this point, the patient may be referred for surgery if videokeratoscopy shows that no corneal distortion remains.

For wearers of RGP lenses with no signs of corneal distortion, lens wear will probably have to be discontinued for no more than a week or two until a normal topographic pattern is found. For soft lens wearers, an even shorter period of discontinuation of lens wear (approximately 1 week) will usually suffice for a normal topographic pattern to be found.

Postoperative Monitoring of Corneal Topography

After RK or excimer laser PRK, corneal topography should be monitored periodically. The goal of excimer laser PRK is to bring about a relative flattening of the area that has been ablated by the excimer laser (usually having a diameter of 5–6 mm), thus reducing the myopia. As described in Chapter 10, during the first few weeks after the surgery there is a *hyperopic shift* due to exaggerated corneal flattening. The hyperopic shift will gradually subside, with the result that the refractive error will stabilize over a period of several months. During this period, the corneal topography will also stabilize.

Among the problems that can be found by videokeratoscopy during the postsurgical period are *irregular astigmatism* and the occurrence of a *central island*. Fortunately, these conditions occur in only very small percentages of patients; when they do occur, however, they can be responsible for a decrease in spectacle-corrected visual acuity. The most common cause of postsurgical irregular astigmatism is *poor centration of the ablated area.* With improvements in surgical procedures, this problem should gradually disappear. A central island is a small area at or near the apex that is *steeper* than the surrounding corneal surface and thus interferes with visual acuity. Although central islands may be seen during the first few weeks or months after surgery, in most cases they are no longer present by several months or a year after surgery.

☼ CLINICAL PEARL

The use of videokeratoscopy is not at all necessary in routine contact lens fitting and may be considered of marginal use in orthokeratology. Videokeratoscopy is a necessary procedure for the comanagement of keratorefractive surgery patients.

References

Bogan SJ, Waring GO, Ibraham O, et al. Classification of normal corneal topography based on computer assisted videokeratography. Arch Ophthalmol 1990;108: 945–949.

Buege T, Hanna R, Grosvenor T. Comparison of corneal topography obtained by keratometry and videokeratoscopy. Int Contact Lens Clin 1996;23:142–148.

Grosvenor T. Clinical use of the keratometer in evaluating the corneal contour. Am J Optom Arch Am Acad Optom 1961;36:237–246.

Grosvenor T. Contact Lens Theory and Practice. Chicago: Professional Press, 1963.

Klyce SD. Computer assisted corneal topography: high resolution graphic presentation and analysis of photokeratoscopy. Invest Ophthalmol Vis Sci 1984;25: 1427–1435.

Lester FS, Harris MG, Keller S, Larsen D. Clinical applications of corneal topography. Int Contact Lens Clin 1994;21:170–174.

Lowther GE. Computerized videokeratoscopy: just pretty pictures or a valuable clinical tool? Int Contact Lens Clin 1994;27:160.

Maeda N, Klyce SD. Videokeratoscopy in contact lens practice. Int Contact Lens Clin 1994;21:163–169.

Maguire LJ. Update on Keratoconus: Insights from Corneal Mapping. In RE Selser (ed), Medical Cornea—Corneal and Refractive Surgery. New York: Kulger, 1994;31–38.

Maguire LJ, Singer DE, Klyce SD. Graphic presentation of computer analyzed keratoscope photographs. Arch Ophthalmol 1987;105:223–230.

Nesburn AB, Hofbauer J, Macy JI. Keratoconus in photorefractive keratectomy (PRK) candidates detected by computer-assisted corneal topography (CAT). Ophthalmology 1992:99(Suppl):126.

Rabinowitz YS, Garbus J, McDonnell PJ. Computer-assisted corneal topography in family members of patients with keratoconus. Arch Ophthalmol 1990;108: 365–371.

Reynolds AE. Corneal topography as found by photoelectronic keratoscopy. Contacto 1959;3:229–253.

Roberts C. The accuracy of "power" maps to display curvature data in corneal topography systems. Invest Ophthalmol Vis Sci 1994;35:3525–3532.

Rowsey JJ, Reynolds AE, Brown R. Corneal topography: Corneascope. Arch Ophthalmol 1981;9:1093–1100.

Rowsey JJ, Balyeat HD, Monlux R, et al. Prospective evaluation of radial keratotomy: photokeratoscope corneal topography. Ophthalmology 1988;95:322–333.

Salmon TO, Horner DG. Comparison of elevation, curvature, and power descriptors for corneal topographic mapping. Optom Vis Sci 1995;72:800-808.

Wilson SE, Lin DT, Klyce SD. Corneal topography of keratoconus. Cornea 1991;10:2–8.

CHAPTER 9

Myopia Control or Reduction with Rigid Contact Lenses

Rigid contact lenses may be used (1) to control the progression of myopia during childhood (using conventionally fitted rigid lenses) and (2) to reduce the existing amount of myopia, usually in adults (using specially designed lenses). The latter procedure is known as *orthokeratology*.

Control of Progression with Conventionally Fitted Rigid Lenses

Practitioners who were involved in contact lens fitting during the 1950s and 1960s, when the only contact lenses available were made of polymethyl methacrylate (PMMA), will recall that many patients were pleased that their lenses lasted longer than glasses. Some young adults who were fitted with contact lenses during their late teen years—when the progression of myopia tends to level off no matter what is done—were convinced that their contact lenses would never have to be made stronger.

Grosvenor (1963) reported seeing a myopic patient who had been wearing "flatter than K" contact lenses and decided to give them up for spectacle lenses. However, he could no longer see well through his spectacle lenses, and it was found that they were approximately 1.50 D too strong. He discontinued wearing his contact lenses for a period of 3 weeks, during which time the cornea gradually steepened and the myopia increased to a point where he could again wear his old glasses. Similar experiences were shared by many practitioners.

Myopia Control with Polymethyl Methacrylate Lenses

In a report published in 1956, Morrison stated that during the previous 2 years he had fitted 1,021 myopes ages 7–19 years with contact lenses, all lenses having posterior curves from 1.62 to 2.50 D flatter than the flattest corneal meridian. He reported in the article that there had been no progression in any of the cases surveyed, and he suggested that the lack of progression was due to a flattening of the cornea, an interference with the metabolism of the cornea, or other factors. In a later report, Morrison (1960) stated that he then used the alignment method of fitting (the back curve being essentially parallel to the flattest corneal meridian) and that he still was finding no progression of myopia.

Of the many case reports and studies of PMMA contact lenses for myopia control, the most convincing was the 5-year case-control study by Stone and colleagues at the London Refraction Hospital (1973, 1976). The experimental group consisted of 84 myopes who were fitted with PMMA contact lenses; the control group consisted of 40 myopes who were fitted with spectacles. The initial ages of the subjects ranged from 6.5 to 16.5 years. Members of the experimental group were fitted with lenses that were "just steeper than the flattest keratometer reading."

On completion of the 5-year study, keratometry and refraction were performed immediately after lens removal. Stone (1976) provided data for 60 eyes of contact lens wearers and 14 eyes of spectacle wearers. The mean increase in myopia was 0.50 D for the contact lens wearers (progression of 0.10 D per year) and 1.75 D for the spectacle wearers (0.35 D per year). The mean change in keratometer readings was a corneal flattening of 0.50 D for the contact lens wearers and a flattening of less than 0.12 D for the spectacle wearers. In discussing these results, Stone made the point that not all of the difference in progression rates for the two groups could be attributed to corneal flattening, "suggesting that there is some retarding effect on axial elongation, but the mechanism is unknown and requires further study." Axial length measurements were not made. In evaluating the results of this study, it should be noted that some members of both the experimental and control groups were as old as 16.5 years—an age at which myopia continues to progress little, if any—when the study began (as shown by Goss and Winkler, 1983).

Do Soft Contact Lenses Control Myopia Progression?

During the 1970s, soft (hydrogel) contact lenses became increasingly popular and, until the development of the rigid gas-permeable (RGP) lens, came close to completely replacing rigid lenses. There was never any evidence that soft contact lenses would be effective in controlling the progression of myopia: On the contrary, soft contact lenses are known to occasionally cause myopia to *increase*, apparently due to corneal edema. On the basis of his private practice data in Canada—at a time when soft lenses were not yet available in the United States—Grosvenor (1975) reported that, for some soft contact lens wearers, myopia increased during the first few months of lens wear, along with corneal steepening. In a review of the records of 120 myopes, ages 24–39 years, who were fitted in his optometry practice, Pence (1992) found that the mean progression of myopia for soft lens wearers was 0.125 D per year. This was approximately 10 times the mean progression for rigid lens wearers, and the mean progression for spectacle wearers fell between these two extremes. On the basis of these and other reports (Horner et al. 1996), we may conclude that soft contact lenses have absolutely no effect in controlling or reducing myopia and, in fact, are more likely to increase the existing amount of myopia.

Myopia Control with Rigid Gas-Permeable Lenses

When RGP contact lenses became available, the question arose as to whether these lenses, like PMMA lenses, would be capable of controlling the progression of myopia. Bailey (personal communication, 1984), a contact lens lecturer and writer, commented that practitioners were recommending the use of RGP lenses not only for the control of myopia progression but also for the reduction of astigmatism in spite of the fact that no definitive studies had been conducted. He suggested that there was a need for such a study.

The Houston Rigid Gas-Permeable Myopia Control Study

In 1985, a 3-year study of the use of RGP contact lenses for myopia control was begun at the University of Houston (Perrigin et al., 1990; Grosvenor et al., 1991a,b). Subjects for the study were 100 myopic children, ages 8–13 years, who were fitted with Paraperm silicone-acrylate RGP lenses (dK = 42) (Paragon Vision Sciences, Mesa, AZ). Criteria for inclusion in the study were at least 1 D of myopia with no more than 2 D of astigmatism, normal binocular vision, normal ocular health, and no history of contact lens wear. A "historical" control group was used, consisting of 39 single-vision spectacle wearers who had served as controls in a previous study of bifocal control of myopia (Grosvenor et al., 1987). The control subjects were matched with the experimental subjects on the basis of initial age and initial amount of myopia.

Most members of the experimental group were fitted with lenses having an overall diameter of 9.0 mm and an optic zone diameter of 7.7 mm. A small number were fitted with lenses having diameters as large as 9.5 mm or as small as 8.5 mm. Secondary and peripheral curve radii and center thicknesses were those normally used by the manufacturer. Lenses were fitted by the alignment method, using the following criteria: an alignment fit as indicated under UV light after instillation of fluorescein, with a complete peripheral ring of pooling and the absence of a stagnant apical pool and a well-centered lens with approximately 2 mm of lag after a blink.

The study was conducted by two teams of researchers: an evaluation team and a patient care team. The evaluation team made baseline measurements consisting of manifest retinoscopy and subjective refraction, keratometry, and ultrasound measurement of the axial distances. These measurements were repeated at yearly intervals for the duration of the study. The testing was done on a Saturday morning before subjects put their lenses on (having worn them on a full-time basis up until the day before the testing was done). Members of the patient care team closely supervised student clinicians in the fitting and follow-up care. Changes in lens power or fitting parameters (base curve, etc.) were made as needed during the course of the study. Members of the evaluation team were unaware of any previous refractive or biometric findings or any of the data collected by the patient care team, but responsible patient care required that members of the patient care team had access to both the evaluation team data and the patient care team data.

Three-Year Results
At the end of the 3-year period, data were analyzed for the right eye of each subject. Of the original 100 subjects, 56 remained in the study. At that time, it was necessary to "rematch" experimental and control subjects, which resulted in a control group of 20 (rather than the original 39) subjects. For the 56 contact lens wearers, the mean progression of myopia was 0.48 D (SD ± 0.70 D) for the 3-year period, or 0.16 D per year, whereas for the control group, the mean progression was 1.53 D (SD ± 0.81 D), or 0.51 D per year (Perrigin et al., 1990). The mean annual progression for each group is illustrated graphically in Figure 9.1. Although the mean progression during the 3-year period was approximately 1.00 D greater for the spectacle wearers than the contact lens wearers, there were large amounts of variation for members of both groups. For the contact lens wearers, the 3-year change in refraction varied all the way from 1.25 D *less myopia* to 2.00 D more myopia, whereas for the spectacle wearers, the 3-year change varied from 0.50 D more myopia to 3.00 D more myopia.

The mean change in corneal power for these 56 subjects was a flattening of 0.37 D (SD ± 0.32 D), and the mean change in axial length was an increase of 0.48 mm (SD ± 0.48 mm). There was a wide distribution in both corneal power change and axial length change. For corneal power, the modal value was *no change*, with some corneas flattening as much as 1.25 D. Axial length changes varied from an apparent decrease (probably due to the experimental error involved in taking the measurements) to an increase of more than 1.0 mm.

On the basis of these 3-year results, Perrigin et al. (1990) arrived at the following conclusions:

1. For wearers of Paraperm RGP contact lenses, myopia progressed at a significantly slower mean rate than for wearers of spectacle lenses. However, *for a given patient* it would not be possible to predict the

FIGURE 9.1. Mean annual progression of myopia for contact lens wearers and spectacle wearers. (Reprinted with permission from J Perrigin, D Perrigin, S Quintero, T Grosvenor. Silicone acrylate contact lenses for myopia control: 3-year results. Optom Vis Sci 1990; 67:765–769.)

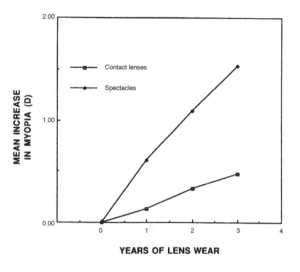

effect of contact lenses on progression, due to the large standard deviations for both groups.

2. The slower rate of progression for the RGP lens wearers was associated with corneal flattening (mean, 0.37 D during the 3-year period).
3. Corneal flattening, as measured by the keratometer, accounted for no more than one-half of the effect of the lenses in controlling myopia progression. A tentative explanation is that the corneal flattening may take place primarily in the apical portion of the cornea, whereas the keratometer measures an annulus having a chord diameter of approximately 3 mm.
4. The results are consistent with the suggestion by Stone (1976) that contact lens wearing may have an effect on axial elongation. This appears to be due to a decrease in anterior chamber depth: Goss and Erickson (1990) showed that a decrease in anterior chamber depth of 0.1 mm due to a backward displacement of the cornea would be responsible for a change in refraction of 0.14 D in the direction of less myopia.

☼ CLINICAL PEARL

When a myopic child is motivated to wear contact lenses, the use of RGP contact lenses is likely to reduce the rate of progression when compared with progression with glasses or soft contact lenses. However, for an individual child it is not possible to predict whether—and to what extent—RGP contact lenses will reduce progression.

Effect of Discontinuation of Lens Wear

An important question when contact lenses are used for myopia control is "What happens when the patient discontinues lens wear?" To answer this

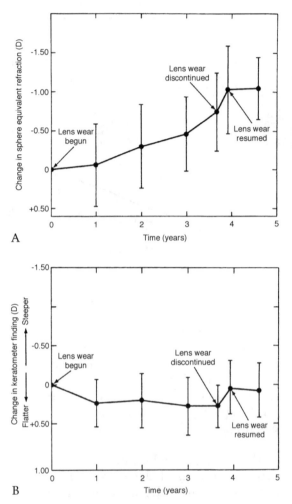

FIGURE 9.2. Graphs showing mean changes (and standard deviations), right eye, for 23 subjects who completed the 44-month study. (A) Spherical equivalent refraction. (B) Keratometer findings. (Reprinted with permission from T Grosvenor, D Perrigin, J Perrigin, S Quintero. Rigid gas permeable contact lenses for myopia control: effects of discontinuation of lens wear. Optom Vis Sci 1991;68: 385–389.)

question, the 56 subjects who completed the 3-year study were invited to continue wearing their lenses until the following summer, and then to discontinue wearing them during the summer vacation. Those subjects who agreed to discontinue lens wear were required to turn in their contact lenses (to make sure that they would not be worn) and were fitted with glasses to be worn during the summer. At the end of the summer, they were fitted with new contact lenses, which they wore during the following school year. Most of the 56 subjects discontinued lens wear during the summer, but only 23 remained in the study by returning to the clinic for the visit at the end of the summer (to be fitted with new contact lenses) and then returning once again for a re-evaluation at the end of the following school year. As shown in Figure 9.2A, during the 10-week period of non-wear, myopia increased by an average of approximately 0.37 D, but there

TABLE 9.1
Summary of the Results of Studies of Myopia Control Using Conventional Rigid
Contact Lenses Fitted by the Alignment Method

	London Study Stone (1976)	*Houston Study Perrigin et al. (1990)*
Type of lens used	PMMA	Paraperm (dK = 42)
Duration of study	5 yrs	3 yrs*
Initial ages of subjects (yrs)		
Experimental	8.5–16.5	8–13
Control	6.5–16.5	8–13
Number of subjects completing the study		
Experimental	60	56
Control	14	39
Mean progression of myopia		
Experimental	0.10 D/yr	0.16 D/yr
Control	0.35 D/yr	0.48 D/yr

PMMA = polymethyl methacrylate.
*Before discontinuing lenses for a 10-week period.

was no further increase during the subsequent 8-month period after lens wear was resumed. Figure 9.2B shows that for these 23 subjects, corneal power decreased by an average of 0.25 D during the more than 3 years of contact lens wear, increased back to the original value during the 10 weeks of nonwear, and then flattened slightly after lens wear was resumed.

It was concluded by Grosvenor et al. (1991a) that in spite of the fact that the contact lenses were discontinued for the 10-week period, the total progression during the more than 4.5-year period was no greater than would have been expected if lens wear had not been discontinued. The mean progression during the entire period (0.99 ± 0.83 D) was significantly less than would have been expected if glasses rather than contact lenses had been worn for the entire period (1.90 ± 0.81 D).

The results of these PMMA and RGP myopia control studies are shown in Table 9.1. An obvious difference between the two studies is the lower mean progression rate for subjects in the London study, for both spectacle-wearing and contact lens–wearing subjects. This difference is very likely due to the fact (mentioned in the discussion of the London study) that the initial ages of subjects in the London study were as high as 16.5 years—when the progression of myopia would be expected to level off—whereas none of the subjects in the Houston study were older than 13 years when the study began.

☼ CLINICAL PEARL

Any effect that RGP contact lenses have in controlling the progression of myopia for a given wearer depends on continued lens wear. If lens wear is discontinued for a relatively short period of time (e.g., a few weeks), myopia progression will probably accelerate. When lens wear is resumed, progression rates will again decrease.

Can We Predict Which Myopic Children Will Benefit by Wearing Rigid Contact Lenses?

Even with PMMA contact lenses, which were often fitted larger and thicker than the currently used RGP lenses, many myopic children continued to progress. I (TG) can report that my own daughter, who began wearing PMMA contact lenses at the age of 8 years, when she had 3.00 D of myopia, continued to progress until the age of 18 years, at which time she had 9.00 D of myopia. And she was a "good" contact lens wearer, wearing her lenses for 12 hours or more per day, and always following instructions concerning hygienic lens care. However, she came from a long line of myopes: Her father, two of her uncles, her two brothers, and several cousins all had moderate or high myopia. This suggests—but does not prove—that rigid contact lenses are less likely to reduce the progression of myopia for children who have a strong genetic background for myopia.

☼ CLINICAL PEARL

In discussing contact lenses for myopia control with parents and their myopic children, practitioners should bear in mind that when myopia "runs in the family" and/or when a child has a relatively large amount of myopia at an early age, the myopia is likely to progress no matter what is done.

Bifocal Rigid Gas-Permeable Contact Lenses for Myopia Control

Because bifocal spectacle lenses have been shown to control the progression of juvenile myopia—particularly in the presence of nearpoint esophoria or a high lag of accommodation (Goss, 1986; Goss and Grosvenor, 1990)—and because RGP contact lenses have also been shown to control the progression of juvenile myopia (Perrigin et al., 1990; Grosvenor et al., 1991a,b), it is reasonable to expect that bifocal RGP contact lenses might have an even greater effect in controlling myopia. This method of myopia control has been suggested to the authors by Hom (personal correspondence, 1997).

As this book goes to press, almost no information is available concerning the efficacy of this method of myopia control. In the one report we have been able to find, wearing Conforma VFL-3 aspheric "nonbifocal bifocal" contact lenses (Conforma Laboratories, Norfolk, VA) stabilized a teenager's myopia as well as her nearpoint esophoria. Hansen (1997) reported his results on a 13-year-old myopic girl who presented with 5Δ of nearpoint esophoria. After wearing single-vision RGP contact lenses for one year, the patient's myopia progressed only 0.25 D (from –2.00 to –2.25 D), but the nearpoint esophoria increased to 16Δ. At this time, Softperm (combination

RGP and soft) contact lenses (Wesley Jessen, Des Plaines, IL) were prescribed, and during the following year the myopia progressed approximately 2 D and the nearpoint esophoria increased to 22Δ. Conforma VFL-3 aspheric multifocal RGP contact lenses were then prescribed, with the result that during a period of 4 years, there was no significant myopia progression, and the nearpoint esophoria had reduced to 14Δ through the distance portions of the lenses and to orthophoria through what was described as the "+2.00 D effective add power."

Orthokeratology with Conventionally Designed Rigid Lenses

Orthokeratology may be defined as the procedure in which rigid contact lenses are fitted in such a way as to flatten the corneal apex and thus reduce or eliminate the existing myopia. Orthokeratology had its beginnings during the 1960s, when PMMA contact lenses were purposely fitted much flatter than the conventional "alignment" fit, with the intention of reducing or eliminating myopia by flattening the cornea. In the 1980s, when RGP lenses had all but completely replaced PMMA lenses, these lenses too were used by orthokeratologists. Whether PMMA or RGP lenses were used, the lenses were of conventional design with a secondary curve having a radius several millimeters flatter than the base curve. The late 1980s saw the introduction of "reverse geometry" lenses for orthokeratology: The secondary curve of a reverse geometry lens is *steeper*, rather than flatter, than the base curve, with the intention of molding the cornea in such a way that the apex is flattened while the midperiphery is steepened. As this book goes to press, reverse geometry lenses are becoming increasingly popular, although studies demonstrating their long-term efficacy are yet to be published.

Perhaps the earliest suggestion of what was later to be called orthokeratology was that of Jessen (1962), who described what he called the *orthofocus technique*. This was a method of making use of a plano PMMA lens, fitted sufficiently flat so that the correction of the refractive error was brought about entirely by the "tear lens" power. For an eye having 3.00 D of myopia, the base curve of the lens would be fitted 3.00 D (or 0.6 mm) flatter than the flattest corneal meridian, with the expectation that the cornea would eventually flatten to match the curvature of the contact lens and, therefore, contact lenses would no longer be needed. Assuming that the cornea flattened as expected, no changes in contact lens curvature or power would be anticipated.

During the next two decades, numerous methods of orthokeratology were advocated, most of which, unlike Jessen's method, required the sequential fitting of several pairs of contact lenses. Most of these methods required the use of large, thick, relatively flat lenses (although not as flat as advocated by Jessen) with gradually flatter lenses being fitted at predetermined intervals.

Typically, once the cornea flattened by 0.25 or 0.50 D, a flatter pair of lenses was fitted, and this procedure was repeated until no further flattening occurred. At this point, wearing time would be gradually reduced with the aim of having the patient wear the lenses the minimum number of hours per day required to maintain the orthokeratologic effect. "Retainer" lenses were often prescribed to be worn for a certain number of hours each day or to be worn during sleep. The orthokeratology literature during this period consisted almost entirely of descriptions of various practitioners' individual techniques, with little or no evidence concerning results. However, starting in the late 1970s, results of several clinical studies of orthokeratology were reported.

Houston Orthokeratology Study

The results of the first prospective clinical trial of orthokeratology, conducted at the University of Houston, were reported by Kerns (1976, 1977, 1978), who emphasized that he was taking an objective position by not advocating the use of orthokeratology but by investigating it on a scientific but clinically oriented basis. Three groups of subjects were recruited for the study: Thirty-six experimental subjects (ages 12–29 years) were fitted with PMMA lenses designed for orthokeratology; 26 control subjects (ages 13–24 years) were fitted with conventional PMMA lenses; and six control subjects (ages 22–24 years) were fitted with spectacle lenses. Initial refractive errors were –3.50 D or less, with no more than 1.00 D of astigmatism. The 26 contact lens control subjects were fitted by the alignment method, using conventionally designed lenses. The 36 experimental subjects were initially fitted also by the alignment method but with larger, thicker lenses to "initiate" corneal flattening: When corneal flattening began to occur, flatter lenses were sequentially fitted. All six spectacle-wearing controls remained in the study for 700 days, at which time data were available for 14 conventional contact lens–wearing control subjects and 34 orthokeratology subjects. Graphs published by Kerns (1977) showed the following approximate mean changes in refractive error at 700 days:

Spectacle-wearing control subjects: no change

Conventional contact lens–wearing control subjects: 0.25 D less myopia

Orthokeratology subjects: 1.00 D less myopia

In addition, the orthokeratology subjects had a mean of approximately 0.50 D of induced with-the-rule astigmatism, whereas for the conventional contact lens wearers, there was no induced astigmatism. Furthermore, the mean amount of induced with-the-rule astigmatism shown by the orthokeratology subjects varied greatly with time.

Kerns (1977) reported that the limiting factor for inducing corneal flattening was the *sphericalization* of the cornea, which occurs when the corneal apex has become sufficiently flat that its radius of curvature is similar to that of the periphery. He made the point that the standard deviations were so high that it would not be possible to predict the outcome for an individual patient. No data were given concerning the permanency of the orthokeratology changes.

Binder et al. Orthokeratology Study

A masked study of 23 subjects undergoing orthokeratology and 16 control subjects fitted with conventional rigid contact lenses was reported by Binder et al. (1980). Average ages for subjects in the two groups were 23.4 and 21.1 years, respectively. Mean initial refractive errors were -2.42 D for the orthokeratology subjects and -5.00 D for the control subjects. Results were reported in terms of improvement in uncorrected visual acuity rather than reduction of myopia, with 70% of the orthokeratology subjects experiencing 20/40 uncorrected acuity. However, Binder et al. published a graph showing, surprisingly, *a greater mean reduction in myopia for control subjects* than for orthokeratology subjects. At 24 months, when only six control subjects and 12 orthokeratology subjects remained in the study, mean reductions in myopia were 1.75 D for control subjects but only 1.00 D for orthokeratology subjects.

In discussing their results, Binder et al. (1980) stated that when lens wear was discontinued, there was a rapid reduction in visual acuity. They also stated that approximately one-third of the orthokeratology subjects required reading glasses to perform their near activities (the ages of these subjects were not reported) and that "the quality of unaided visual acuity was significantly worse than the best corrected visual acuity obtained with glasses or contact lenses."

Berkeley Orthokeratology Study

In a randomized clinical trial conducted at the University of California at Berkeley (Brand et al., 1983; Polse et al., 1983a,b), 40 orthokeratology subjects and 40 controls were fitted with rigid contact lenses and followed for a period of 18 months. The initial subjects were 20–35 years of age, with myopia from 1 to 4 D and astigmatism of less than 0.75 D. The study was conducted in three phases: phase A, a 2-month adaptive phase; phase B, a 12-month postadaptive phase; and phase C, a 4-month lens withdrawal and postwearing phase. Subjects were randomized into the experimental and control groups, with the result that they did not know which group they were in. "Real" lens changes were made for members of the experimental group, and "mock" lens changes were made for members of the control group. As in the Kerns (1976, 1977, 1978) study, orthokeratology subjects were fitted with larger, thicker, and flatter lenses than the control subjects. PMMA lenses were used initially for all subjects, but Polycon RGP lenses (dK = 12) (Wesley Jessen) were later fitted for 14 orthokeratology subjects and 3 control subjects because of corneal edema and other problems.

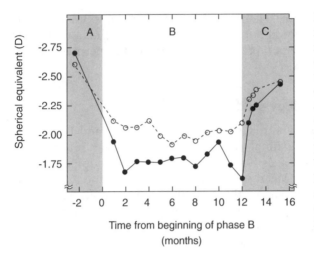

FIGURE 9.3. Graph showing changes in mean spherical equivalent refraction during the three phases of the study, for orthokeratology subjects (solid circles) and control subjects (open circles). (Reprinted with permission from KN Polse, RJ Brand, JS Schwalbe, DW Vastine, R Keener. The Berkeley orthokeratology study. Part II: efficacy and duration. Am J Optom Physiol Opt 1983;60:187–198.)

Means of subjective refraction findings were plotted (reproduced here as Figure 9.3) for the orthokeratology subjects (solid circles) and control subjects (open circles) who completed the study. As shown in this graph, at the end of the 12-month postadaptation phase, the changes in refractive error obtained for the 31 orthokeratology subjects and 28 control subjects remaining in the study were as follows: orthokeratology subjects, a mean decrease in myopia of 1.00 D, and control subjects, a mean decrease in myopia of 0.50 D. As also shown in Figure 9.3, during the withdrawal and postwearing phase the mean refractive error quickly returned to within 0.25 D of the initial mean refractive error for both the orthokeratology and control subjects. Polse et al. (1983a) concluded that the reduction in myopia could be perpetuated only with the use of retainer lenses and that vision was variable from day to day.

Pacific University Orthokeratology Study

Coon (1984) reported on a study conducted at the Pacific University College of Optometry making use of *steep-fitting* PMMA lenses. The reason for using steep-fitting lenses was to avoid the problem of induced corneal astigmatism that often occurs when flat-fitting lenses are used for orthokeratology. The 80-week study initially involved 24 orthokeratology subjects and 15 control subjects who wore conventional PMMA contact lenses. Subjects in both groups had myopia between 1 and 3 D with keratometer findings between 41 and 46 D, and had little or no previous contact lens wear. Mean ages were 26.9 years for the control subjects and 24.4 years for the orthokeratology subjects.

The Tabb method of fitting was used for both the experimental and control subjects. Coon (1984) described this method as being based on a *theoretical tear reservoir*, which he defined as "the percentage of the posterior lens surface occupied by the intermediate and peripheral curve area." Using this method, for a given overall diameter, the theoretical tear reservoir (%) is manipulated by changing the optic zone diameter. For the control subjects, a 30% tear reservoir was maintained for the duration of the study; however, for the experimental subjects, the tear reservoir was initially 32.5%, and was increased by increments of 2.5% to a maximum of 45%. This was done by keeping the overall diameter of the lens constant and decreasing the optic zone diameter, which has the effect of gradually loosening the fit of the lens without creating a "flat" fit.

At the end of the 80-week period, 14 subjects remained in the experimental group, and eight subjects remained in the control group. The mean reduction in spherical equivalent myopia differed little for the two groups, being 0.58 D for the experimental group and 0.46 D for the control group. Corneal topography was monitored by use of the Photo-Electronic keratoscope (Wesley Jessen), and it was found that, for both the experimental and control groups, the corneas became less aspheric, on average, approaching a spherical profile, which had also been reported by Kerns (1977) but only for experimental subjects.

The results of orthokeratology studies making use of conventional rigid contact lenses are summarized in Table 9.2. As shown in this table, the most convincing studies were those of Kerns (1976, 1977, 1978) and Polse et al. (1983a): In both these studies, the mean decrease in myopia was 1.00 D for experimental subjects and was at least twice the mean decrease in myopia for control subjects. In addition, these two studies made use of much larger groups of subjects than the other two studies.

☀ CLINICAL PEARL

The use of sequentially flatter-fitting conventionally designed rigid contact lenses for orthokeratology may provide a clinically significant advantage as compared with the use of these lenses when fitted by the usual alignment method. However, it is not possible to predict the result for a given patient, and maintenance of the effect depends on the routine use of retainer lenses.

Accelerated Orthokeratology with Reverse Geometry Lenses

With the availability of silicone-acrylate and fluoro-silicon-acrylate rigid lens materials, oxygen permeability was sufficiently high so that lenses no longer had to be fitted loosely enough for the cornea to receive most of its oxygen supply through "tear pumping" (the pumping of tears from under the lens, with each blink). Wlodyga and Bryla (1989) suggested that RGP contact lenses for orthokeratology should be made *steeper* in the intermediate zone, rather than flatter, for the following reasons: (1) Such a "reverse geometry" lens would cause the midperiphery of the cornea to steepen,

TABLE 9.2
Summary of the Results of Orthokeratology Studies Using Conventionally
Designed Rigid Contact Lenses Fitted Flatter than the Corneal Optic Zone

	Kerns (1976–1978)	Binder et al. (1980)	Polse et al. (1983a)	Coon (1984)
Type of lens used	PMMA	PMMA	PMMA[a]	PMMA
Duration of study	2 yrs[b]	2 yrs[b]	14 mos[c]	80 wks
Initial ages of subjects (yrs)				
Experimental	12–19	Av 23.4	20–35	Av 24.4
Control	13–28	Av 21.1	20–35	Av 26.9
Number of subjects completing study				
Experimental	34	12	31	14
Control	14	6	29	8
Mean reduction in myopia (spherical equivalent)				
Experimental (D)	1.00	1.00	1.00	0.58
Control (D)	0.25	1.75	0.50	0.46

Av = average; PMMA = polymethyl methacrylate.
[a]PMMA lenses were used initially for all patients, but Polycon lenses (dK = 12) were later fitted for 14 orthokeratology subjects and three control subjects because of edema and other problems.
[b]Some subjects were followed for longer periods of time, but 2 yrs was taken as the cut-off point for the sake of comparison and because large numbers of subjects dropped out in the later months.
[c]The duration of the study was 18 mos, but data were reported at the end of the post–wearing phase of the study.

while the optical zone flattens; (2) the lens design would allow better control over centration, reducing the resulting astigmatism; and (3) orthokeratology changes would occur much more quickly. Following the Wlodyga and Bryla suggestion, Nick Stoyan of Contex, Inc. (Sherman Oaks, CA) developed the *Contex OK* series of lenses, using a material having a dK of 88. Other reverse geometry lenses currently available are the *Plateau* lens (Menicon Co. Ltd., Clovis, CA) and the *RK/Bridge* lens (Conforma). The claim has been made that reverse geometry lenses are twice as effective in causing "ortho-K" changes as conventional rigid lens designs, with the result that when these lenses are used the procedure is known as *accelerated orthokeratology*.

Fitting the Contex OK Lenses

Wlodyga and Bryla (1989) suggested the following patient selection criteria for accelerated orthokeratology with the Contex OK lens: (1) myopia up to 6 D; (2) no previous rigid lens wear; (3) keratometer power from 40 to 46 D; (4) no more than 3 D of corneal cylinder; (5) ability to wear a Contex OK lens with reasonable comfort; (6) 15–40 years of age; and (7) no pathology. In addition, they suggested that a "temporal K" reading should be taken (in the horizontal meridian only) by instructing the patient to look nasally and fixate on the "+" sign of the Bausch & Lomb Keratometer mire (Bausch & Lomb, Rochester, NY). If the temporal horizontal reading is flatter than the central horizontal reading, "the chances of flattening the central cornea are excellent."

The three basic lenses in the Contex OK series are the OK-2, the OK-3, and the OK-4. All three lenses have a posterior optic zone diameter of 6.0 mm, a steeper intermediate curve, and a flatter aspheric periphery; however, they differ in that the posterior intermediate curve is 2 D, 3 D, and 4 D steeper, respectively, than the posterior optic zone. The OK-3 is typically used as the initial lens; the OK-4 is used if additional apical flattening is desired; and the OK-2 is often used as a retainer lens. The most often used overall diameter for the OK-3 lens is 9.8 mm, but larger or smaller diameters may be used. The OK-5P lens, like the OK-3, has a secondary curve 3 D steeper than the optic zone, but differs from the OK-3 by having a 6.5-mm optic zone diameter and by incorporating 1–3Δ of base-down prism, to aid in achieving centration. The OK-6 and OK-7 lenses have 6.5- and 7.0-mm diameters, respectively. The intermediate curve steepening differs for the two lenses, being 2.5 D for the OK-6 and 2 D for the OK-7.

In fitting the OK lenses, the base curve of the first lens is routinely ordered 1.00–1.50 D (0.20–0.30 mm) flatter than the flattest corneal meridian. The expected fluorescein pattern shows apical touch surrounded by an annulus of fluorescein pooling under the steep intermediate curve which, in turn, is surrounded by an area of bearing under the aspheric peripheral curve. Soni and Horner (1994) suggest that the first lens order should consist of three or four pairs of lenses, each subsequent pair being 0.50 D (0.10 mm) flatter than the previous pair and having a refracting power 0.50 D less than the previous pair. They suggest that follow-up visits be scheduled:

4 hours after dispensing

3 days after dispensing

1 week later

An additional week later

Biweekly visits for the first 3 months

After successful myopia reduction, every 3–6 months

During follow-up visits, the fit of the lenses is carefully monitored with regard to the apical touch, the width of the annulus of fluorescein pooling (the tear reservoir), and the adequacy of tear exchange. When the cornea begins to flatten, the entire lens will fit closer to the cornea, indicating that a lens with a flatter base curve is needed.

Use of Retainer Lenses

All candidates for orthokeratology should be told that once the desired reduction in myopia has been achieved, there is a high probability that the use of retainer lenses will be necessary to maintain adequate unaided visual acuity. In discussing retainer lenses, Mountford (1997) has made the following suggestions:

1. If the unaided visual acuity, refractive error, or corneal topography shows no alteration over two consecutive monthly visits, the treatment phase of orthokeratology is considered complete, and the retainer phase commences. By this stage, the patient is expected to have attained uncorrected acuity of 6/6 (20/20) with approximately 0.50 D of hyperopia. Because the aim of orthokeratology is to correct vision to the stage at which constant contact lens wear is no longer necessary, overnight lens wear is the logical solution to the problem.

2. Once the retainer lenses have been designed, they are worn on an all-waking-hours schedule for 1 week, and the results are assessed. At this point, if the visual acuity and refraction are acceptable, the patient is advanced to the extended-wear program of 7 days and 6 nights for the next few weeks or months to stabilize the induced corneal changes.

3. When these changes have stabilized, the wearing schedule for retainer lens wear is based on the length of time the patient retains acceptable visual acuity after lens removal on awakening in the morning: When vision blurs, the lenses are reinserted and worn until the next morning.

4. As for the design of the retainer lenses, Mountford (1997) suggested that, if the patient fails to achieve 20/20 acuity when the cornea and refractive error have stabilized, the last set of OK lenses becomes the retainers. It the cornea and refractive error have not stabilized, he suggested a number of options for retainer lenses, including OK lenses (avoiding steep base curves and small optic zones) and custom-designed conventional contour or aspheric lenses.

Results with Accelerated Orthokeratology

As this chapter is being written, case reports concerning accelerated orthokeratology are appearing in the vision care literature; unfortunately, reports of long-term retrospective or prospective clinical studies are conspicuous by their rarity.

Case Reports

Wlodyga and Bryla (1989) reported what they called their "best case results." The patient was a 4-year wearer of extended-wear soft lenses whose myopia was progressing. Before being fitted with Contex OK lenses, the patient's refraction and keratometer readings (central and temporal) were the following:

R   –4.50 –1.25 x 155; corrected VA 20/20; CK 42.25/42.50 @090; TK 40.62

L   –4.00 –1.50 x 060; corrected VA 20/20; CK 42.00 DS; TK 40.37

During a period of 7 weeks, the patient wore four pairs of OK lenses, each pair having a flatter base curve radius and lower minus power than the preceding pair. At the end of the 7 weeks, the refraction and keratometer findings were the following:

R   Uncorrected VA 20/25; –0.50 DS; CK 39.75/43.37 @090; TK 41.37

L   Uncorrected VA 20/15; Plano; CK 39.75/43.37 @090; TK 43.50

At this point, the patient was fitted with retainer lenses to be worn 8 hours per day. The authors did not comment on the more than 3 D of induced with-the-rule corneal astigmatism and its effect (or lack of effect) on visual acuity. (As already mentioned, induced with-the-rule corneal astigmatism is likely to occur with high-riding lenses.)

Horner and Bryant (1994) reported on a 28-year-old male who needed a minimum of 20/200 uncorrected acuity in each eye as a job requirement. His uncorrected visual acuity, refractive error, and central keratometer findings were the following:

R   Uncorrected VA 20/400; –3.75 –0.75 x 180; CK 44.75/45.00 @090

L   Uncorrected VA 20/400; –2.50 –1.75 x 175; CK 44.37/46.75 @085

Contex OK-3 lenses were dispensed, having base curves 2.00 D flatter than the central keratometer reading for the right eye and 1.50 D flatter for the left eye. After wearing these lenses for only 4 hours, uncorrected acuity improved to right eye 20/200 and left eye 20/60, with a decrease in myopia of 0.50 D for the right eye and 1.00 D for the left eye. During the next 2 months, three more pairs of lenses were dispensed. The final pair had base curves of 40.37 D for the right eye and 39.75 D for the left eye (4.37 D and 4.62 D flatter than the original central keratometer readings in the flat meridian). The patient was examined after wearing the final lenses for a period of 1 year, at which time his uncorrected acuity was right eye 20/40 and left eye 20/30. The daily wearing time during the 1-year period was not reported.

In their book *Orthokeratology Handbook*, Winkler and Kame (1995) published several case reports. In one of these reports, the patient was a 24-year-old man whose myopia had been progressing while wearing soft contact lenses. His prefitting uncorrected acuity, refraction, and keratometer findings were the following:

R   Uncorrected acuity 20/200; –2.00 DS; CK 44.62/44.75; TK 41.75

L   Uncorrected acuity 20/200; –2.00 DS; CK 44.75 DS; TK 41.75

The following OK-3 lenses were ordered (note that the *tear lens power* for each eye, with these lenses, is –1.50 D):

R   –0.50 D, base curve 7.83 mm (43.12 D); diameter 9.6 mm

L   –0.75 D, base curve 7.80 mm (43.25 D); diameter 9.6 mm

The day after the dispensing visit, when the lenses had been worn a total of 10 hours, the findings were the following:

R   Uncorrected acuity 20/100; –1.25 –0.25 x 180; CK 44.50/44.75; TK 41.75

L   Uncorrected acuity 20/200; –1.50 DS; CK 44.75 DS; TK 41.75

During the next several weeks, three additional pairs of lenses were ordered, each being flatter and having less minus (or more plus) power than the previous pair. The fourth pair of lenses did not center well, so the third pair of lenses was used as retainer lenses to be worn on a split schedule, 2 hours each in the morning and evening. The third pair had the following prescription:

R   +0.25 D, base curve 8.01 mm (42.12 D); diameter 10.0 mm

L   +0.25 D, base curve 7.99 mm (42.25 D); diameter 10.0 mm

After 1 month of wearing the retainer lenses, uncorrected visual acuity was R 20/25, L 20/20-1. Because the control of myopia progression was one of the patient's main goals, +0.75 D adds in the form of spectacles were prescribed for reading.

Retrospective and Prospective Studies

In a review of the records of 126 patients fitted with Contex OK-3 lenses by Dr. Dwight Cooper in Evansville, Indiana, Horner et al. (1992) reported their results in the form of four graphs (reproduced here as Figure 9.4) showing the time course of myopia reduction during 6 months of orthokeratology treatment based on the initial amount of myopia. As shown in Figure 9.4, after 6 months of treatment, the mean reductions in myopia (±SD), based on the initial amount of myopia, were the following:

FIGURE 9.4. Graph showing time course of myopia reduction during the first 6 months of orthokeratology treatment using Contex reverse geometry lenses for four groups of subjects based on initial amount of myopia. (Reprinted with permission from DG Horner, WH Wheeler, PS Soni, DR Gerstman, GG Heath. A noninvasive alternative to radial keratotomy. Ophthal Vis Optics Tech Dig 1992;3:42.)

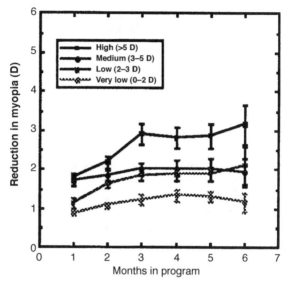

Initial Myopia	Eyes	Mean Reduction
Less than –2.00 D	56	1.00 ± 0.50 D
–2.00 to –3.00 D	54	1.75 ± 0.75 D
–3.00 to –5.00 D	56	2.00 ± 0.75 D
Greater than –5.00 D	60	2.25 ± 1.25 D

In a discussion of the Evansville results, as well as the results obtained with the Contex OK lenses on patients fitted at the Indiana University School of Optometry, Horner and Bryant (1994) concluded that orthokeratology using the Contex OK-3 lens appears to reduce myopia by at least 2 D in most patients and that this technique appears to reduce myopia by approximately twice the amount of previous methods and in half the time. They warned, however, that significant chair time is required for this procedure and that at least one out of four patients will drop out due to discomfort, inadequate myopia reduction, or other problems.

☼ CLINICAL PEARL

Results with reverse geometry lenses for accelerated orthokeratology show that these lenses have approximately twice the effect of "standard geometry" RGP lenses when used for orthokeratology, which, in turn, have approximately twice the effect of conventionally fitted RGP lenses in reducing myopia or controlling myopia progression. As with standard geometry RGP lenses, when reverse geometry lenses are used, retainer lenses are almost always necessary to maintain acceptable visual acuity.

Mountford's Fitting Method

Mountford (1997) criticized the fitting method outlined in the Contex fitting manual, pointing out that "it totally depends on the practitioner's ability to assess the fluorescein pattern accurately, which with such a radical lens design and so many variations requires both a high degree of skill and experience." He concluded that a more accurate and predictable approach is required. Mountford's method is based on the combination of corneal sag, tear layer thickness, and lens sag as integral factors in the calculations used to design lenses "that show predictable fitting characteristics." He provided a formula for calculation of the corneal sag, based on information concerning corneal curvature and eccentricity obtained by the use of corneal topography systems such as the EyeSys and TMS instruments, together with a formula used for computer-generated calculations of the sag of Contex OK lenses.

As an example, Mountford's computer program indicates that for a cornea having an apical radius of 7.80 mm and an eccentricity (at a chord of 8.80 mm) varying from 0.30 to 0.60, a Contex lens should have an optic zone width of 6.0 mm and an optic zone radius varying from 8.20 to 8.35 mm, whereas the Contex rule of thumb would indicate, for all eccentricities, an optic zone radius 0.30 mm flatter than the apical radius of the cornea, or 8.10 mm. He made the point that the rule-of-thumb lens would result in a tight lens unless the corneal eccentricity was on the order of zero. Although not mentioned by Mountford, this represents an interesting challenge because very few corneas have an eccentricity of zero. A cornerstone of the use of reverse geometry lenses is that for orthokeratology to be successful, the greater the eccentricity (in other words, the flatter the corneal periphery as compared with the corneal apex), the better.

Mountford (1997) described a retrospective study of 23 patients, comparing the Contex rule-of-thumb method and his calculation method. Group 1, consisting of 13 patients, had been fitted by the Contex method (0.30–0.40 mm flatter than the apical corneal radius), whereas group 2, consisting of 10 patients, had been fitted by the calculation method (0.30–0.65 mm flatter than the apical corneal radius). For each patient, the change in corneal power after 6 hours of lens wear was determined, using the subtractive plot function of the EyeSys.

Group 1 patients were found to have a mean decrease in corneal power of 0.91 D (SD = 0.36 D), and group 2 patients were found to have a mean decrease in corneal power of 1.38 D (SD = 0.58 D). Using analysis of variance, the difference was found to be significant ($p = .0024$, $F = 10.373$). However, no information was provided concerning corneal flattening for the two groups of patients beyond the initial 6 hours of wear, and no information was provided concerning matching of the patients in the two groups in terms of refractive error, age, or other factors.

Role of Videokeratoscopy
in Accelerated Orthokeratology

As noted in Chapter 8, corneal curvature changes occurring in accelerated orthokeratology can be monitored either by a combination of central and peripheral keratometry or by videokeratoscopy. Changes in central corneal curvature can obviously be monitored by the use of a standard keratometer, and peripheral corneal changes can be monitored, to some extent, by the simplified form of peripheral keratometry in which readings are taken while the patient fixates, in turn, the two plus signs and the two minus signs of the keratometer mire. Advantages of this latter procedure are that it is possible to determine when *sphericalization* has taken place—that is, when the cornea is no flatter in the periphery than at the apex—and it is possible to determine whether the curvature changes are taking place in a symmetrical manner, which will occur if lens centration is adequate. However, if more detailed information concerning the corneal contour is desired, the use of videokeratoscopy may be advantageous.

Accelerated Orthokeratology Compared
with Refractive Surgery

Accelerated orthokeratology by the use of reverse geometry lenses has often been described as a noninvasive alternative to refractive surgery. Horner et al. (1992) reported that they had used videokeratoscopy to compare 20 eyes that had undergone orthokeratology with 12 eyes that had undergone radial keratotomy (RK) surgery and 14 normal, unaltered eyes. Before gathering the videokeratoscopy data, they observed that most orthokeratology patients had nearly spherical post-treatment refractive errors and very good unaided visual acuity, whereas RK patients reported reduced acuity through spectacles, and some complained of glare and unstable vision. On the basis of the videokeratoscopy data, Horner et al. examined the mean radii of curvature, in 0.2-mm steps from the center of the cornea. The unaltered corneas showed a fairly stable curvature within a 2-mm annulus at the corneal apex, and a steady flattening toward the periphery. The orthokeratology corneas were not significantly different than the normal corneas out to approximately a 3-mm radius, but just a little flatter. The RK corneas varied significantly from the normal and orthokeratology corneas, showing a flattening out to an annulus having a 1-mm radius and then a steepening at each annular step to a maximum at a 3.2-mm radius.

In another study, Soni and Horner (1994) plotted the reduction in myopia against the original amount of myopia for three sets of data: (1) retrospective orthokeratology data (described above) from an optometric practice in Evansville, Indiana; (2) data from orthokeratology patients fitted with Contex OK lenses at Indiana University; and (3) 1-year RK data resulting from the PERK (Prospective Evaluation of Radial Keratotomy) study. Their graph is reproduced here as Figure 9.5. Soni and Horner con-

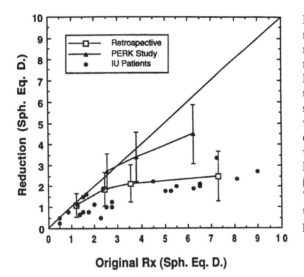

FIGURE 9.5. Comparison of myopia reduction with Contex reverse geometry lenses and radial keratotomy (Prospective Evaluation of Radial Keratotomy [PERK] study). (Rx = prescription; IU = Indiana University; Sph. Eq. D. = spherical equivalent diopters.) (Reprinted with permission from PS Soni, DG Horner. Orthokeratology [Chapter 49]. In ES Bennett, BA Weissman [eds], Clinical Contact Lens Practice. Philadelphia: Lippincott, 1994;1–7.)

cluded that orthokeratology using the Contex OK lenses produces twice the myopic reduction of that shown with flat-fitting conventional PMMA or RGP lenses, and approximately 60% of the reduction produced by RK as reported in the PERK study.

The results of orthokeratology and RK were compared in a study by Lakin et al. (1995). Their study included five subjects who had undergone orthokeratology and five who had undergone RK. All subjects were 22–29 years of age, with spherical equivalent refractive errors ranging from –2.25 to –4.37 D. Subjects in the two treatment groups were matched as closely as possible for refractive errors. The authors published graphs showing the initial and final spherical equivalent refractive errors for each of the 10 subjects. Interpretation of these graphs indicates that the mean final refractive error (right eye) was –0.80 D for the RK subjects (range, –0.50 to –1.00 D) and –0.75 D for the orthokeratology subjects (range, –0.25 to –1.00 D); the mean reduction in myopia for both the RK and orthokeratology subjects ranged from approximately 1.75 D for initial myopia of –2.25 D to approximately 3.00 D for initial myopia of –4.37 D. Lakin et al. concluded that both orthokeratology and RK are effective in reducing myopia and astigmatism and that most patients were happy with the final unaided visual acuity and experienced no deleterious effects.

Phillips (1995) compared accelerated orthokeratology and laser photorefractive keratectomy (PRK) and stated what he considered to be the advantages and disadvantages of both procedures. Among the points made by Phillips are the following:

1. Orthokeratology is reversible; PRK is not.
2. PRK causes permanent corneal changes; orthokeratology does not.

3. The long-term effects of orthokeratology are known to be safe, but the long-term effects of PRK are unknown.
4. Visual acuity remains optimal with orthokeratology, but not necessarily with PRK.
5. PRK involves pain; orthokeratology involves adaptational irritation only.
6. Prescription changes are easily made in orthokeratology by changes in retainer design, but changes in PRK require further ablation.
7. Orthokeratology requires tolerance of RGP wear, whereas many PRK patients are contact lens failures.
8. Orthokeratology requires ongoing contact lens wear, but at least half of PRK patients require no optical aid.
9. PRK is more successful than orthokeratology for high amounts of myopia.

Phillips did not, however, compare the *adverse effects* of the two procedures. Whereas adverse effects of orthokeratology are absent or minimal, possible adverse effects of PRK surgery (see Chapter 10) include a reduction in best-corrected visual acuity, regression of the surgical effect (myopic drift), poor vision in low-contrast situations, poor vision in the presence of glare, and problems with night driving.

☼ CLINICAL PEARL

For myopia in the −1.00 to −3.00 D range (which includes the great majority of myopic eyes), accelerated orthokeratology with reverse geometry lenses can bring about a reduction in myopia that compares favorably with the reduction brought about by RK. Except in very rare cases of extremely low amounts of myopia, retainer lenses will have to be worn to perpetuate the orthokeratology effect.

Orthokeratology after Refractive Surgery

As discussed in Chapter 10, a high percentage of patients who have undergone keratorefractive surgery, such as RK or PRK, will eventually find that they must wear glasses or contact lenses for distance vision, near vision, or both. This is particularly true of RK, because *hyperopic drift* has been shown to take place for as long as 10 years after the surgery (Waring et al., 1994). This problem is exacerbated by the fact that many people who undergo RK are at an age when they will soon become presbyopic or are already presbyopic.

Wlodyga (1992) reported on a patient who had undergone RK surgery with the hope of attaining uncorrected acuity of 20/40 in the poorer eye to qualify as a fireman. Preoperatively, he was a 9.00 D myope with corrected acuity of 20/20, each eye; however, 8 months after the RK surgery his residual refractive error and unaided acuity were the following:

R   –2.00 DS, 20/60

L   –3.00 DS, 20/200

Contex OK-9 lenses (10.5 mm overall diameter, 6 mm optic zone, base curve 8.70 mm, secondary curve 6 D [1.2 mm] steeper than base curve) were fitted to be worn 8 hours per day. On the second day, the lenses had become too tight and were replaced by OK-9 lenses having 8.90 base curves. Within 6 weeks, unaided acuity was right eye 20/20 and left eye 20/40. At this time, he was fitted with 10.0-mm diameter aspheric periphery lenses to be worn at night, which maintained "functional unaided acuity for the rest of the day." Wlodyga suggested that "we orthokeratologists should let our ophthalmologic friends know that we are able and willing to apply our skills in contact lens fitting to help our patients have more satisfactory results."

Note on the Legal Status of Reverse Geometry Lenses

As this book goes to press, the legal status of reverse geometry lenses in the United States is unclear. Approval by the U.S. Food and Drug Administration (FDA) is normally given only for lens materials—not for lens designs—and the materials used in the Contex OK lens and other reverse geometry lenses have been given FDA approval. However, it is our understanding that manufacturers of reverse geometry lenses have, so far, not applied for FDA approval of the lens design, which obviously differs greatly from that of "standard-geometry" RGP lenses. This lack of FDA approval of reverse geometry lens designs could possibly be considered as an "off-label" use of the approved lens materials, which might prove to be a problem for practitioners as well as for manufacturers.

References

Binder PS, May CH, Grant SC. An evaluation of orthokeratology. Ophthalmology 1980;87:729–744.

Brand RJ, Polse KA, Schwalbe JS. The Berkeley orthokeratology study, part I: general conduct of the study. Am J Optom Physiol Opt 1983;60:175–186.

Coon LJ. Orthokeratology, part II. Evaluating the Tabb method. J Am Optom Assoc 1984;55:409–418.

Goss DA. Effect of bifocal lenses on the rate of childhood myopia progression. Am J Optom Physiol Opt 1986;63:135–141.

Goss DA, Erickson P. Effects of changes in anterior chamber depth on refractive error of the human eye. Clin Vis Sci 1990;5:197–201.

Goss DA, Grosvenor T. Rates of myopia progression with bifocals as a function of nearpoint phoria: consistency of three studies. Optom Vis Sci 1990;67:637–640.

Goss DA, Winkler RL. Progression of myopia in youth: age of cessation. Am J Optom Physiol Opt 1983;60:651–658.

Grosvenor T. Contact Lens Theory and Practice. Chicago: Professional Press, 1963.

Grosvenor T. Changes in corneal curvature and subjective refraction of soft contact lens wearers. Am J Optom Arch Am Acad Optom 1975;52:405–413.

Grosvenor T, Perrigin J, Perrigin D, Quintero S. Houston myopia control study, a randomized clinical trial. 2. Final report by the patient care team. Am J Optom Physiol Opt 1987;64:482–498.

Grosvenor T, Perrigin D, Perrigin J, Quintero S. Rigid gas permeable contact lenses for myopia control: effects of discontinuation of lens wear. Optom Vis Sci 1991a;68:385–389.

Grosvenor T, Perrigin D, Perrigin J, Quintero S. Do rigid gas permeable contact lenses control the progression of myopia? Contact Lens Spectrum 1991b;5:29–35.

Hansen DW. Bifocal RGP lenses for progressive myopia. Contact Lens Spectrum 1997;11(10):15.

Horner DG, Bryant MK. Take another look at today's ortho-K. Rev Optom 1994; 131(6):43–46.

Horner DG, Soni PS, Salmon TO, Schroeder T. Junior high age children's myopia progression in soft lenses vs. spectacles (abstract). Invest Opthalmol Vis Sci 1996;37:S1004.

Horner DG, Wheeler WH, Soni PS, et al. A noninvasive alternative to radial keratotomy. Ophthal Vis Optics Tech Dig 1992;3:42.

Jessen GN. Orthofocus techniques. Contacto 1962;6:200–204.

Kerns RL. Research in orthokeratology. Parts I–VIII. J Am Optom Assoc 1976;47: 1047–1051, 1275–1285, 1505–1515; 1977;48:227–238, 345–359, 1124–1147, 1541–1543; 1978;49:308–314.

Lakin D, Estes S, Carter W. Reshaping your ideas. Contact Lens Spectrum 1995; April:25–30.

Morrison R. Contact lenses and the progression of myopia. Optom Weekly 1956;47: 1487–1488.

Morrison R. The use of contact lenses in adolescent myopic patients. Am J Optom Arch Am Acad Optom 1960;37:165–168.

Mountford J. Orthokeratology. In AJ Phillips, L Speedwell, J Stone, T Hough (eds), Contact Lenses (4th ed) Boston: Butterworth–Heinemann, 1997;653–692.

Pence N. Effect of contact lenses on myopic progression in 24–39 year olds. Optom Vis Sci 1992;69(Suppl):72.

Perrigin J, Perrigin D, Quintero S, Grosvenor T. Silicone acrylate contact lenses for myopia control: 3-year results. Optom Vis Sci 1990;67:765–769.

Phillips AJ. Orthokeratology—an alternative to excimer laser? J Br Contact Lens Assoc 1995;18:65–71.

Polse KN, Brand RJ, Schwalbe JS, et al. The Berkeley orthokeratology study. Part II: Efficacy and duration. Am J Optom Physiol Opt 1983a;60:187–198.

Polse KN, Brand RJ, Keener R, et al. The Berkeley orthokeratology study. Part III. Safety. Am J Optom Physiol Opt 1983b;60:321–328.

Soni PS, Horner DG. Orthokeratology. In ES Bennett, BA Weissman (eds), Clinical Contact Lens Practice. Philadelphia: Lippincott, 1994.

Stone J. Contact lens wear in young myopes. Br J Physiol Opt 1973;28:90–134.

Stone J. The possible influence of contact lenses on myopia. Br J Physiol Opt 1976;31:89–114.

Waring GO, Lynn MJ, McDonnell PJ. Results of the Prospective Evaluation of Radial Keratotomy (PERK) study 10 years after surgery. Arch Ophthalmol 1994;112:1298–1308.

Winkler TD, Kame R. Orthokeratology Handbook. Boston: Butterworth–Heinemann, 1995.

Wlodyga RJ. Orthokeratology: a case in point. How do you handle the post-RK patient? Contact Lens Spectrum 1992;7(12):28–32.

Wlodyga RJ, Bryla C. Corneal molding: the easy way. Contact Lens Spectrum 1989;4(8):58–65.

CHAPTER 10

Keratorefractive Surgery

Numerous keratorefractive surgical procedures have been devised not only for myopia but also for aphakia, hyperopia, and astigmatism. Procedures currently in use for the management of myopia include radial keratotomy (RK), laser photorefractive keratectomy (PRK), automated lamellar kerato-plasty (ALK), laser in situ keratomileusis (LASIK), and intrastromal corneal ring (ICR) implantation.

Radial Keratotomy

Almost 50 years ago, RK was introduced by Sato et al. (1953), who made use of radially oriented incisions in both the anterior and posterior surfaces of the cornea with the purpose of flattening the cornea's optic zone and thus reducing or eliminating myopia. Unfortunately, the incisions in the posterior cornea tended to cause severe edema, with the result that the procedure was soon abandoned.

Radial keratotomy was reintroduced by Fyodorov and Durnev (1979), who reported that they used 16 radial incisions in the anterior corneal sur-face, to a depth of three-fourths of the corneal thickness, on 60 eyes of 30 patients having preoperative myopia from –0.75 to –3.00 D. In all cases, the central corneal curvature flattened by 5–6 D within a few days after surgery and then began to stabilize. After Fyodorov and Durnev's report, many oph-thalmic surgeons traveled to Russia to learn the procedure, with the result that RK rapidly became a popular form of myopia management in this coun-try. As reported in the AOA News (July 1, 1980), however, the National Eye Advisory Council "expressed grave doubts" concerning the procedure, which was being adopted on a large scale even though there was not an adequate basis on which to assure the public of its safety and efficacy.

Waring and coworkers conducted a multicenter study of RK called the Prospective Evaluation of Radial Keratotomy, or PERK, study. The study was designed to investigate the safety, efficacy, predictability, and stability of a

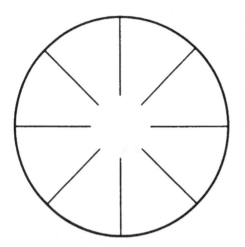

FIGURE 10.1. Radial keratotomy, consisting of eight equally spaced incisions made deeply in the corneal stroma to flatten the central cornea. (Reprinted with permission from GO Waring. Making sense of "Keratospeak." A classification of refractive corneal surgery. Arch Ophthalmol 1985;103:1472–1477.)

single, standardized surgical technique of RK. Subjects for the study were 435 patients, 21–58 years of age, having bilateral physiological myopia from –2.00 to –8.00 D, and refractive astigmatism no greater than 1.50 D. The surgical procedure involved eight radial incisions (Figure 10.1), providing a clear optic zone of 3.0, 3.5, or 4.0 mm, depending on the amount of preoperative myopia. Radial keratotomy was initially done on only one eye of each subject.

One year after surgery, Waring et al. (1985) reported that the percentage of patients having a spherical equivalent refractive error within ±1.00 D of emmetropia varied from 84% for subjects having preoperative myopia between –2.00 and –3.13 D to only 38% for patients having preoperative myopia between –4.25 and –8.00 D. The percentage of patients having unaided visual acuity of 20/20 varied from 71% for the low myopes to only 26% for the high myopes.

Evaluation of Radial Keratotomy

Postoperative problems with RK range from complaints of glare and fluctuating vision, which are relatively common, to traumatic rupture and keratitis, which fortunately occur only rarely. However, the problems that have received the most attention are poor predictability of refractive outcome, a high prevalence of postoperative anisometropia, loss of best-corrected visual acuity, the postoperative need for glasses or contact lenses, and a persistent hyperopic drift.

Glare and Fluctuating Vision

Reports of glare are common in situations such as night driving when the pupils are dilated. Fluctuating vision—due to a diurnal variation in corneal power and refractive error—is also a relatively common complaint. In a study of 46 patients who complained of fluctuating vision 1 year after undergoing RK, Schanzlin et al. (1986) reported a mean increase in myopia of 0.42 D, a mean corneal steepening of 0.42 D, and a mean visual acuity loss of approximately one line of letters between 7 and 8 AM and 7 and 8 PM. More recently, Bullimore et al. (1994) reported that 10 firefighters who had undergone RK had visual acuity that met the firefighter standard at 8 AM, but three failed to meet the standard at 3:30 PM. As a result, they suggested that when a visual acuity standard is required of applicants for employment who have undergone RK, the standard should be amended to include visual acuity testing both in the early morning and late afternoon.

Predictability of Refractive Outcome

As already noted, 1-year PERK study results showed that relatively small percentages of patients achieved uncorrected visual acuity of 20/20 or were within ±1.00 D of emmetropia. Moreover, there is no way to predict *which* patients will achieve 20/20 acuity or a near-plano refractive error.

Loss of Best-Corrected Visual Acuity

Myopes who have undergone RK surgery are likely to make comments such as "Since my surgery, I see much better without glasses than I did before, but I don't see as well with my glasses." In the 1-year PERK study report, Waring et al. (1985) noted that 13% of eyes had lost one or two lines of best-corrected visual acuity. This acuity loss can be devastating for a person whose occupation or avocation requires precise visual acuity. Thus, it is not surprising that relatively few refractive surgeons—many of whom are myopic—have personally undergone RK surgery.

Postoperative Anisometropia

In the 3-year PERK study results, Waring et al. (1987) reported that 41% of the patients who had undergone RK surgery in both eyes had anisometropia of 1.00 D or more. This is a prevalence more than four times greater than that for adults who have not undergone keratorefractive surgery. Duling and Wick (1988) have reported four cases of significant binocular vision difficulties associated with anisometropia resulting from RK.

Need for Glasses or Contact Lenses

Although the purpose of RK is to make the use of corrective lenses unnecessary, follow-up PERK study reports showed that relatively high percentages of patients were wearing glasses or contact lenses. Bourque et al. (1994) reported that 6 years after surgery, of the 328 patients who returned a questionnaire, 48% were wearing glasses or contact lenses on a part-time or full-time basis: 17% for distance vision, 15% for near vision, and 16% for both distance and near vision. For 374 patients who were examined 10 years after surgery, Waring et al. (1994) reported that glasses or contact lenses were worn—for distance or near vision or both—by 36% of patients younger than 40 years of age and by 67% of patients older than 40 years of age.

Hyperopic Drift

That so many of the PERK study patients needed glasses for reading 6 years and 10 years after surgery was due mainly to two factors: (1) Many of these patients were initially presbyopic or had become presbyopic since the surgery was performed, and (2) a long-continued hyperopic drift occurred for many patients. Ten-year data for the PERK study (Waring et al., 1994) showed a mean hyperopic drift of almost 1 D. Dietz et al. (1994) reported that for 42 patients who had reported for all examinations during a postoperative period averaging 8.5 years, mean hyperopic drift was 1.26 D, from a mean spherical equivalent refraction of +0.56 D at 1 year to +1.82 D at 8.5 years.

Discussing this hyperopic drift, Lindstrom (1997) said, "Those of us who performed radial keratotomy in the 1980s have created a significant number of hyperopes. . . . The average radial keratotomy patient was 35 to 40 years old; now they are 45 to 50, presbyopic, potentially hyperopic, and unhappy."

Postoperative Traumatic Injury and Keratitis

The literature on RK includes several reports of postoperative traumatic injury and keratitis. Forstot and Damiano (1988) reported on a series of seven cases of post-RK trauma. In three of these cases, the trauma was due to a tennis ball; in one case the trauma was due to a tire iron; in one case it was due to a war-game pellet; and in two cases, it was due to leaning over and striking the globe with a solid object. Simmons et al. (1988) reported that a patient had suffered a ruptured globe when struck in the eye by an elbow on the twenty-fourth day after uneventful RK surgery. In spite of surgical repair, the blind, painful eye had to be enucleated. The authors suggested that all patients undergoing RK surgery should be advised to use protective eyewear, but they noted that this would defeat the purpose of RK surgery, which is to avoid the encumbrance of eyewear.

Mandelbaum et al. (1986) reported that three patients had developed keratitis 7–30 months after uncomplicated RK surgery. In all three cases, ulcers developed along the keratotomy scars. With treatment, all three cases healed without a reduction in visual acuity. Shivitz and Arrowsmith (1986) described two cases of delayed keratitis, developing 9–45 months after RK surgery. In one case, the causative organism was found to be *Pseudomonas aeruginosa*, and in the other case both *Staphylococcus* and *Moraxella* species were found. Both patients responded to treatment and regained 20/20 acuity.

☼ **CLINICAL PEARL**

Patients who seek advice concerning RK surgery should be informed of the possibility that glasses or contact lenses may still be needed for distance vision, near vision, or both and that if glasses are worn, "corrected" vision may not be as clear as it was before the surgery. They should be told of the problems that may occur postoperatively, including glare and fluctuating vision, and the remote possibility of a serious eye injury due to the weakened condition of the globe.

Innovations in Radial Keratotomy Surgery

During the years that have elapsed since the first PERK study report in 1985, many improvements have taken place in RK surgery. These improvements involve the use of shorter and fewer incisions and the use of incisions designed to correct astigmatism.

The Casebeer System

The system advocated by Casebeer (1997) not only uses shorter (and sometimes fewer) incisions than were used in the PERK study, but also approaches the problem of predictability by being biased toward an *undercorrection*—minimizing the possibility of overcorrection—with the result that one or more enhancement procedures may be undertaken if necessary. Using this system, the diameter of the clear zone varies from 3.25 to 5.00 mm, depending on the amount of the desired correction and the number of incisions, and the incisions spare the limbus by ending at an 8-mm optic zone. Because eyes of older patients show a greater effect for the same number of incisions and clear-zone size, Casebeer makes use of a nomogram that takes into consideration not only the desired correction and number of incisions, but also the patient's age.

According to Casebeer (1997), approximately 35–40% of patients undergo enhancements: An enhancement is considered "only if the patient's vision is worse than 20/40 uncorrected, if there is significant and symptomatic anisometropia, or if the patient desires further improvement." He suggests telling older people that they will be giving up some of their reading ability if they seek an enhancement.

Mini-Radial Keratotomy

Lindstrom (1997) developed what he called "Mini-RK," with the idea of maximizing corneal flattening with the minimum number and length of incisions to stay below the range where the cornea destabilizes. Using this system, the outward extensions of the radial incisions are confined to a zone of 7 mm rather than extending close to the limbus as in conventional RK. For a 3-mm clear zone, this means that incisions are only 2 mm long. Lindstrom presented 3-year data showing a mean hyperopic shift of only 0.04 D (for 72 eyes) from 6 months to 3 years after surgery.

Procedures for Correcting Astigmatism

There is general agreement that, for a myopic eye having no more than 1.00 D of refractive astigmatism, no special "cuts" in addition to the radial incisions need be made. However, for myopic eyes having more than 1.00 D of astigmatism, special procedures for the correction of astigmatism, such as the use of transverse "T-cuts" and arcuate-cuts (as described above for the Casebeer system), are often used. These cuts are centered on the steeper of the two principal meridians.

Fitting Post–Radial Keratotomy Patients with Contact Lenses

Optometric care for post-RK patients is complicated not only by the fact that people who undergo RK do so to get rid of glasses or contact lenses, but also by the fact that many patients who opt for RK have been unsuccessful contact lens wearers. In a discussion of post-RK contact lens fitting, Ebling (reported by Sposato, 1987) commented that fitting these patients requires the practitioner to be an "amateur psychologist": Patients tend to be ecstatic after RK surgery because they think that they will never have to wear glasses again, but then they may seek refractive error correction after approximately 1 year. Although he has had no problems with soft lenses for post-RK eyes, Ebling normally fits rigid gas-permeable lenses for daily wear. He made the following recommendations:

1. The presurgical keratometry readings (which will be several diopters steeper than the postsurgical readings) should be used.
2. A large, Korb-type lens should be used to achieve lateral centration.
3. Due to the steep lens-cornea relationship, the power of the lens will have to be about the same as the power needed to correct the refractive error before surgery.
4. The fluorescein pattern, which will show apical clearance, should be used to evaluate lens fit.
5. Adequate lens movement should be present to ensure tear pumping.
6. Heavy bearing on transverse incisions should be avoided.

☀ CLINICAL PEARLS
Vision care practitioners should expect patients who have undergone RK surgery to be reluctant to wear glasses or contact lenses, in spite of poor visual acuity, asthenopia, or other problems due to the undercorrection or overcorrection of their myopia. When RGP contact lenses are fitted, the presurgical K readings and spectacle prescription should be used as a starting point.

Ethical and Legal Issues

In an editorial in the *Journal of the American Optometric Association*, Vinger (1996), who referred to himself as "one of the 90 percent of ophthalmologists who don't engage in RK surgery," discussed a number of ethical and legal problems regarding RK, including (1) the problem of glare and its effect on night driving, (2) the probable decrease in best-corrected visual acuity, (3) the problem of progressive hyperopia, and (4) the possibility of postoperative rupture of the globe. He commented that he loves his own moderate myopia and that hyperopic patients his age are miserable. As a result of a literature review and conversations with his colleagues, Vinger knew of 30 cases of traumatic ruptured globe through the RK incisions, occurring as late as 10 years after surgery. As an advocate of injury prevention and the use of protective eyewear, he asked how he could justify weakening the eye. He concluded by saying, "I believe that encouraging people to remove properly prescribed protective eyewear and expose themselves to increased risk of eye rupture both is unethical and has the potential of significant legal misfortune. I'll pass on RK, thank you."

Laser Photorefractive Keratectomy

Due to the problems experienced with RK during the 1980s—in particular, its poor long-term predictability—many refractive surgeons were in a position to welcome a surgical procedure that might promise better predictability. Excimer laser surgery was such a procedure.

As described by Marshall (1989), the excimer laser is a chamber in which an inert gas (argon) combines, under extreme pressure and high voltage, with a halogen (fluorine). Once the argon-fluoride molecule is formed, it breaks up and emits an extremely high-energy photon of ultraviolet radiation having a wavelength of 193 nm. The pulse duration of the emitted laser radiation is approximately 10–20 ms, and the pulses are emitted at a rate of 1–100 per second. Commenting that carbon-carbon bonds of human tissue require an energy of three electron volts "to keep them together," Marshall stated that the individual 193-nm laser photon has an energy of 6.4 electron volts, sufficient to cause any biologic macromolecule that absorbs it to literally fall apart—a process known as *photoablation.*

At a seminar sponsored by Summit Technology (Waltham, MA) and The Ohio State University College of Optometry, Marshall (1994) described the process of photoablation by saying that when the laser beam penetrates the corneal tissue, 95% of the energy is absorbed, and broken-up molecules are expelled from the corneal surface at twice the speed of sound, making a crackling sound and a burnt-tissue smell and emitting fluorescence. After the ablation, a pseudomembrane forms over the totally sterile wound, and is the surface on which the epithelial cells come back postoperatively.

As described by L'Esperance et al. (1989), the 10 × 20-mm laser beam is expanded by the use of prisms to a 20 × 20-mm rotating beam. The rotating beam is passed successively through a series of apertures mounted in one of three aperture wheels—one for myopia, one for hyperopia, and one for astigmatism. The aperture wheel used for myopia has a series of apertures of increasing diameter. The ablation profile for myopia is shown in Figure 10.2, to an exaggerated scale, before regrowth of the epithelium. Because each ablation step removes only 0.25 μm of tissue, the ablated surface is smooth to optical standards.

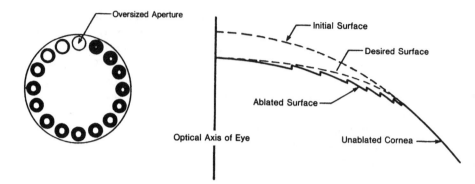

FIGURE 10.2. The aperture wheel used for myopia allows the laser beam to ablate the central cornea more deeply than the peripheral cornea. The diagram on the right shows an exaggerated representation of the stepped profile ablation of the cornea to reduce myopia. (Reprinted with permission from FA L'Esperance, JW Warner, WB Telfair, et al. Excimer laser instrumentation and technique for human corneal surgery. Arch Ophthalmol 1989;47:131–139.)

The Surgical Procedure and the Healing Process

At the Summit Technology seminar, Rejpal (1994) described the PRK treatment procedure. After instillation of a miotic (30 minutes before surgery) and a topical anesthetic, the patient is positioned under helium-neon aiming beams; oriented to the fixation target (a green light within a red ring); and told about the snapping sound, the smell, and the fluorescence that will occur with the photoablation. A speculum is inserted, and the patient is given practice in fixation—which is *very* important: A drop of methylcellulose is placed on the cornea, and the laser beam is delivered on the layer of methylcellulose while the patient fixates the green light. This procedure is repeated, for additional practice, after which the methylcellulose is removed and the beam is delivered to the corneal epithelium to acquaint the patient with the snapping sound. The laser is programmed for the desired correction and for the desired optic zone (usually 6.0 mm), the cornea is marked (in a circle 1 mm larger than the desired optic zone), and the epithelium is removed with a beaver blade, after which the cornea is cleaned to remove epithelial debris. The patient is again instructed concerning fixation, and the laser beam is delivered. The time required for the treatment varies from 13 seconds for a –3.00 D correction to 23 seconds for a –6.00 D correction.

Immediately after surgery, an antibiotic is instilled, the eye is patched, and oral pain medication is administered. After 24 hours, the patch is removed and visual acuity is checked. After 3 days, in most cases the epithelium fully covers the ablated area, and the patient is more comfortable.

The *corneal haze* that occurs after PRK surgery as a part of the healing process was described by Barr (1994). He made the point that the patient is less concerned than the practitioner about the corneal haze,

FIGURE 10.3. The hyperopic shift that occurs during the first few months after laser photorefractive keratectomy surgery, reversing to form a stable refraction. (Reprinted with permission, from print supplied by J Barr. Seminar sponsored by Summit Technology and The Ohio State University College of Optometry. Chicago, August 1994.)

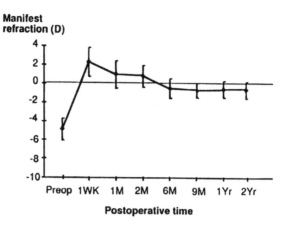

which is due to backward scatter. The corneal haze is related to the healing process, and is graded as follows:

Grade 1	Trace	Slow healing response
Grade 2	Mild	Optimal healing
Grade 3	Moderate	Aggressive healing
Grade 4	Major	More aggressive healing

The haze is related to a postoperative hyperopic shift, shown in Figure 10.3: the greater the haze, the more quickly the hyperopic shift reverses toward a stable refraction. In the great majority of cases, the haze is either *mild* or *moderate*, but in *trace* corneal haze, an extended hyperopic shift usually occurs.

The Summit Technology Study

Barr (1994) described the 12-month results of the Summit Technology PRK phase III Food and Drug Administration (FDA) premarket approval study. The study involved 701 eyes of subjects between 21 and 65 years of age, with a mean age of 37 years. Preoperative refractive errors ranged from –1.50 to –6.50 D, with astigmatism no greater than 1.50 D. As required by the FDA, the second eye was not operated until 6 months after the first eye was operated. The optic zone size was 4.5 mm for one-third of the subjects, and 5.0 mm for the other two-thirds.

Re-epithelialization occurred within 3 days for 91% of the subjects and by 1 week for all subjects. At the end of 1 year, uncorrected acuity was 20/20 or better for 66% of eyes and 20/40 or better for 91% of eyes; residual refractive error was within ±0.50 D of the predicted amount for 54% of subjects and within ±1.00 D of the predicted amount for 77% of subjects. These results are compared with the 1-year results of the PERK study and the 1-year results of the Ruiz et al. LASIK study (described in the following section) in Table 10.1.

TABLE 10.1
Comparison of 1-Year Results of the Waring et al. PERK Study of RK, the Barr
Summit Technology Study of PRK, and the Ruiz et al. Bogata Study of LASIK

	RK *Waring et al.* *(1985)*	PRK *Barr* *(1994)*	LASIK *Ruiz et al.* *(in preparation)*
Number of eyes	435	701	171
Ages of subjects (yrs)	21–58	21–65	Not reported
Initial refractive errors (D)	–2.00 to –8.00[a]	–1.50 to –6.50[a]	–0.25 to –18.25[b]
Initial refractive astigmatism (D)	≤1.50	≤1.50	Mean, 1.15
Residual refractive error			
Within ±0.50 D	22%[c] to 57%[d]	54%	91%
Within ±1.00 D	38%[c] to 84%[d]	77%	98%
Uncorrected acuity: 20/20 or better	26%[c] to 71%[d]	66%	67%

PERK = Prospective Evaluation of Radial Keratotomy; RK = radial keratotomy; PRK = photorefractive keratectomy; LASIK = laser in situ keratomileusis.
[a]Spherical equivalent refraction.
[b]Spherical component or prescription.
[c]For subjects with the highest preoperative amounts of myopia (–4.25 to –8.00 D).
[d]For subjects with the lowest preoperative amounts of myopia (–2.12 to –3.13 D).

Evaluation of Laser Photorefractive Keratectomy

Whereas the performance of RK does not require the use of a device and therefore did not require approval by the FDA, laser PRK *does* require the use of a device and requires FDA premarket approval. This approval is granted, by the FDA's Division of Ophthalmic Devices, in three phases: Phase I consists of data on a small number of nonfunctional (blind) eyes; phase II involves 100–200 subjects to establish the safety and efficacy of the procedure; phase III involves 500–700 subjects to provide further data on safety and efficacy and to provide a database concerning the risks and benefits of the procedure. During 1996, both the Summit (Summit Technology) and VISX (VISX, Santa Clara, CA) excimer lasers were granted FDA approval, but the laser PRK studies reported before that time—with the exception of premarket studies such as the phase III Summit Technology study described above—were all carried out in other countries. In most of these studies, either the Summit or the VISX instrument was used.

Predictability of Postoperative Refractive Error and Visual Acuity

The results of a large number of studies show that the predictability of PRK, in terms of postoperative refractive error and visual acuity, is rela-

TABLE 10.2
Achieved Photorefractive Keratectomy Corrections 18 Months Postoperatively
as Related to Attempted Correction for 60 of the 120 Eyes Whose Data Were
Reported in Graphs Published by Gartry et al. (1992)

Preoperative Refraction (mean) (D)	Eyes	Ablation Depth (mm)	Ablation Width (mm)	Attempted Correction (D)	Achieved Correction	
					Mean (D)	Range (D)
–2.10	20	17	4	–2.00	–2.00	–0.50 to –3.00
–7.13	20	33	4	–5.00	–3.75	–1.00 to –7.75
–10.26	20	44	4	–7.00	–4.00	0.00 to –9.00

Source: Data from S Gartry, MG Kerr Muir, J Marshall. Excimer laser photorefractive keratectomy—18-month follow-up. Ophthalmology 1992;99:1209–1219.

tively satisfactory for low and moderate amounts of myopia, but falls off rapidly for myopia greater than approximately –6.00 D. For example, in a study conducted in London, making use of the Summit laser, Gartry et al. (1992) found that the postoperative refractive error 1 year after surgery was within ±1.00 D of the attempted correction for 95% of a group of 20 eyes having mean preoperative myopia of –2.10 D, reducing to 20% for 20 eyes having mean preoperative myopia of –10.26 D. In the same study, 55% of the –2.10 D group of eyes had postoperative unaided acuity of 20/20 or better, reducing to 0% for the –10.26 D group.

The use of the excimer laser to correct large amounts of myopia presents a challenge to the surgeon in terms of ablation depth and optical zone width: Too deep an ablation and/or too wide an optic zone may not only weaken the cornea structurally but also may make more likely the possibility of a *steep central island*—a steeper island 2–3 mm in diameter within the flatter, ablated area—or other corneal topographic problems. In the Gartry et al. (1992) study referred to above, the optic zone width was 4.0 mm for all eyes, whereas ablation depth varied from 17 μm for eyes having the smallest amount of preoperative myopia to 44 μm for eyes having the largest amounts of myopia. Table 10.2, based on the data shown in graphs published by Gartry et al., shows (last three columns) that for the higher amounts of myopia the *achieved correction* was not only much less than the *attempted correction*, but also the range of achieved corrections increased markedly with the amount of the attempted correction. Although the range of achieved corrections was only 2.50 D for the –2.10 D group, it was 8.00 D for the –10.26 D group.

Loss of Best-Corrected Visual Acuity

Most large-scale studies show that best-corrected visual acuity (compared with best-corrected acuity preoperatively) for many eyes tends to be

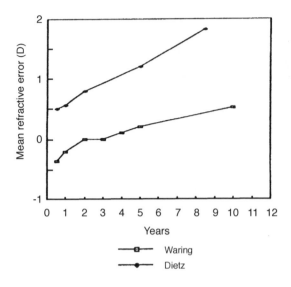

FIGURE 10.4. Mean post–radial keratotomy refractive error during a period of 8.5 years, based on data reported by Dietz et al. (1994), and during a 10-year period, based on data reported by Waring et al. (1994).

reduced during the first weeks or months after surgery but in most cases returns to the preoperative level by the end of a year or longer. In a premarket approval study conducted in Los Angeles by Maguen et al. (1994) involving 59 eyes having preoperative myopia ranging from –1.00 to –7.75 D, the percentage of eyes having an acuity loss of two or more lines of letters was 20% one month after surgery, reducing to 4% at 12 months and 0% at 36 months. In the Gartry et al. (1992) study of 120 eyes having refractive errors from –2.10 to –10.26 D, 12 months after surgery 15% of eyes had a best-corrected acuity loss of one-half or one line of letters, and 4% had a loss of two or more lines of letters. Among the causes of a temporary loss of best-corrected acuity are postoperative corneal haze and scarring; causes of longer-term acuity loss include the presence of a steep central island and a decentered optical zone. The latter problem is due to poor fixation by the patient during the delivery of the laser beam, which is usually due to inexperience or lack of patient training on the part of the surgeon.

Regression of Surgical Effect (Myopic Drift)

Contrary to the situation with RK, in which there is a persistent progression of the surgical effect causing a hyperopic drift, in PRK there is a regression of the surgical effect causing a myopic drift. The hyperopic drift that occurs after RK is illustrated in Figure 10.4, for both the 10-year PERK study data (Waring et al., 1994) and for 8.5-year data reported by Dietz et al. (1994). The myopic drift occurring after PRK is shown in Figure 10.5, based on data reported by Epstein et al. (1994), Kim et al. (1994), Maguen et al. (1994), and Gartry et al. (1992). These curves appear to show that the myopic drift levels off by the eighteenth or twenty-fourth postsurgical month.

FIGURE 10.5. Mean refractive errors after photorefractive keratectomy, showing regression of the surgical effect with time, based on data reported in Epstein et al. (1994), Kim et al. (1994), Maguen et al. (1994), and Gartry et al. (1992). For the Gartry et al. subjects, attempted surgical corrections for the 3 groups of subjects were –2.00 D, –3.00 D, and –5.00 D.

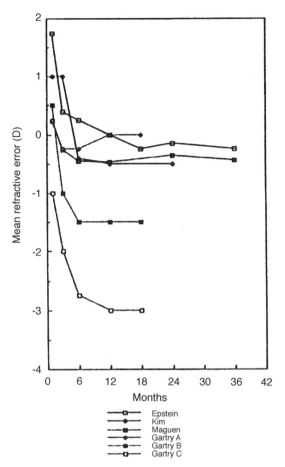

There is no general agreement as to the cause of the myopic drift. Brancato et al. (1993) speculated that the greater regression for the higher myopes may have been caused by an insufficient initial hypercorrection (i.e., the surgical procedure did not bring about a sufficiently high hyperopic shift). Ditzen et al. (1994) concluded that ablation depth—being greater for larger amounts of myopia—is the main factor causing the regression. Until the cause of the myopic drift is understood and corrected, it is not likely that PRK will fully correct myopia greater than approximately –6.00 D. Toward this end, ablation widths have gradually increased, and multistep ablations are being used.

Effects on Vision Other Than High-Contrast Visual Acuity

Even though the result of a PRK procedure may be emmetropia with 20/20 "refracting room" acuity, there are circumstances in which the patient's vision is inferior to his or her preoperative vision with glasses or contacts.

Vision in Low Contrast

Lohman et al. (1991) measured visual acuity at contrast levels of 100%, 20%, and 5% before PRK surgery and for a 12-month period after surgery. Postoperative acuity at 100% contrast was diminished initially—when corneal haze was at its greatest—but returned to preoperative levels after 3 months and remained so throughout the 12-month period. At the 20% contrast level, acuity was slightly lower than at 100% contrast throughout the 12-month period. At the 5% contrast level, the authors stated that "most patients had significant problems with the test during the immediate postoperative period and many could not even see the test letter."

As reported by Black (1997), Casson, a psychophysicist at the Ottawa General Hospital Eye Institute, suggested that refractive surgeons should make use of low-contrast acuity tests (in addition to the usual high-contrast tests) to assess their patients' postoperative vision. In a study of 58 eyes of 48 patients undergoing PRK surgery, Casson found that although high-contrast acuity returned to preoperative levels, performance on low-contrast acuity charts was still poor at 12 months. She recommended the use of low-contrast charts that make use of Snellen letters and therefore provide results that can be compared with the high-contrast acuity. We couldn't agree more! When only high-contrast acuity is tested—particularly when 20/40 is the criterion for success—practitioners tend not to believe a patient who complains about his or her vision.

☼ CLINICAL PEARL

Vision care practitioners should have on hand—and should routinely use—a simple-to-administer variable contrast acuity test making use of Snellen letters, such as the Pelli-Robson or Regan letter charts. The results of low-contrast acuity testing can provide very important information not only for patients who have undergone refractive surgery but also for many other groups of patients, including contact lens wearers and older patients, who may have problems such as dry eyes, incipient cataracts, or age-related macular degeneration.

Vision in Glare

Visual acuity in the presence of glare was measured by Seiler et al. (1994) on 193 eyes of 146 patients who had undergone PRK. One year after surgery, losses of two or more lines of "glare acuity" were found for none of the eyes with corrections up to 3.00 D but were found for 5% of eyes with corrections between 3.00 and 6.00 D and for 43% of eyes having corrections greater than 9.00 D. The authors concluded that because all of the corneas were clear, the glare effect for the more myopic eyes was due to heterogeneity of the postoperative cornea. They commented that most patients with reduced glare vision reported subjective glare at night under dim lighting, but excellent vision under daytime conditions.

Night Vision Problems

Gimbel et al. (1993) distributed a questionnaire to 52 patients who had undergone bilateral PRK surgery. The average follow-up time was 15 months for the first eye and 8 months for the second eye. Of the 42 patients who returned the questionnaire, 90% said they were satisfied with the results of the surgery. However, in answers to specific questions, 60% reported seeing rings or halos at night; 45% reported that "detail of vision is compromised by haze"; 30% reported seeing rays of light; 21% reported symptoms of "scattered light"; and 7% reported seeing multiple images. When asked about vision in various lighting conditions, 64% of respondents reported a reduced quality of vision in dim illumination compared with daylight; 38% reported poorer vision in artificial light than in daylight; and 50% reported difficulties with night driving. The mean age of those who responded was 26.2 years, which is many years earlier than the onset of night-driving problems—due to conditions such as cataracts, dry eyes, and age-related macular degeneration—experienced by drivers who have not undergone refractive surgery.

Ben-Sira et al. (1997) surveyed 173 patients who had undergone PRK surgery at least 1 year previously. In response to a question concerning night driving after surgery, 42 patients said that night driving was a little worse than before surgery, and 14 said that it was much worse. Of the 51 patients who had surgery performed on just one eye, 25 said that they declined to have it performed on the second eye because they were dissatisfied with the results of the surgery on the first eye.

In an editorial titled "Keratorefractive surgery, success, and the public health," Maguire (1994) made the point that the cornea is normally trouble-free but that it is no longer trouble-free after refractive surgery. He added that the changes in its optical performance are irreversible: Once done, there is no return to the preoperative state. He asked the question, "Why worry about refractive surgery as a potential public health hazard when everyone is happy and basking in success?" He answered the question by saying that it is difficult for keratorefractive procedures to generate a regular optical surface over a large enough corneal surface to avoid aberrations in the central field and even more difficult to prevent aberrations in the peripheral visual field.

☼ CLINICAL PEARL

Patients who are interested in undergoing PRK surgery should be told that although their postoperative daytime vision may be adequate, their vision in low-contrast situations and glare may not be good, and their night vision may be so poor that night driving may be a serious problem.

Intraocular Pressure after Photorefractive Keratectomy Surgery

The importance of intraocular pressure (IOP) and visual field measurements before PRK surgery was stressed by Dello Russo (1997), who reported that 1 month after successful PRK surgery, a 55-year-old man complained that "he didn't seem to get enough light in his eye" and was found to have a severe superior visual field defect. There were no records of IOP measurement or visual field testing at any time before the PRK surgery. Dello Russo warned that visual field testing should always be performed before PRK surgery and that practitioners should be aware that IOP readings after PRK surgery in high myopia are probably inaccurate.

In another report, Chatterjee et al. (1997) stated that the lower postoperative pressure readings were due primarily to a reduction in corneal thickness occurring with the PRK surgery—particularly due to the loss of Bowman's layer—and secondarily to corneal flattening. They suggested that surgeons and optometrists should be aware that to determine the true IOP after PRK surgery, a correction using the following regression equation must be added to the IOP measured by tonometry:

$$\text{IOP drop} = 1.6 - (0.4 \times \text{preoperative spherical equivalent refraction})$$

The authors warned that if this practice is not followed, significant increases in IOP (e.g., due to postoperative steroid therapy) may be overlooked and sight-threatening glaucoma may go undetected. They also suggested that "a strong family history of glaucoma, any ocular hypertension, or suspicion of glaucoma should be considered a relative contraindication for PRK because post-PRK measurements of IOP may be unreliable."

Innovations in Photorefractive Keratectomy Surgery

Innovations in PRK surgery that have taken place during the latter part of the 1990s include scanning beam excimer lasers and transepithelial PRK ablation. Both of these procedures are so new that several months or even years will have to elapse before their results can be compared with the established long-term results of "conventional" PRK surgery.

Scanning Beam Excimer Laser

As opposed to the method used by the two broad-beam excimer lasers that have been granted FDA approval—both of which make use of iris diaphragms to control beam width—a scanning beam laser uses a small, fixed beam that scans across the cornea in a programmed manner. McDonnel (1997) stated that scanning beam lasers cause a smaller acoustic shock wave than wide-beam lasers, and provide a relatively smoother ablation. He reported that in the phase II results of the LaserSight LaserScan 2000 (LaserSight, Orlando, FL), at 3 months, 92% of eyes had 20/40 acuity and 71% had 20/25 acuity;

however, by 6 months, some regression had occurred, with the result that only 83% of eyes had 6/12 (20/40) acuity and 61% had 20/25 acuity.

Transepithelial Photorefractive Keratectomy Ablation

Johnson (1997) described a procedure known as *transepithelial multipass multizone PRK*. Rather than using a beaver blade to remove the epithelium manually before using the excimer laser, the epithelium is removed by the initial pass of a wide-beam excimer laser, resulting in "total removal of the epithelium so that you do not obtain any significant change in Bowman's membrane curvature at the end of the epithelial removal." Advantages of this procedure cited by Johnson are less pain, quicker re-epithelialization, less inflammation and haze, and better patient acceptance. In addition, he stated that decentration does not occur, there is very little regression, and "we have virtually eliminated central islands."

☼ CLINICAL PEARL

As is the case with RK, vision care practitioners should become acquainted with the surgeons in their geographic area who perform PRK surgery and should speak frankly with them concerning procedures, success rates in terms of postoperative refractive error and visual acuity, and complications.

Automated Lamellar Keratoplasty

ALK is a modern version of a procedure developed during the 1960s by Barraquer, which he called *keratomileusis* (carving the cornea). A microkeratome is placed on the eye by means of a suction ring, and a predetermined thickness of the cornea—epithelium, Bowman's layer, and superficial stroma—having a diameter of approximately 7 mm is sliced off but remains attached to the cornea by means of a flap. The microkeratome is then used a second time to flatten the cornea by a predetermined amount, and this stromal tissue is discarded. The superficial corneal flap is replaced, and healing occurs without the necessity of sutures. Because this procedure does not require a device, FDA approval is not required. ALK may be used for eyes having myopia greater than 6 D, for which RK and PRK are only partially successful.

Manche and Maloney (1996) reported retrospective ALK data on 135 eyes of 91 consecutive patients 19–57 years of age. For 52 eyes for which 6-month results were available, only 35% were corrected to within ±1.00 D of emmetropia, and 8% had uncorrected acuity of 20/20 or better. One eye lost three lines of best-corrected acuity (from 20/25 to 20/40).

Somewhat more encouraging results were reported by Lyle and Jin (1996), who published 1-year results of a prospective study of ALK on 128 eyes of 81 consecutive patients. The mean age of the patients was 36.6 years, with a range from 20 to 54 years; preoperative refractive errors ranged from a spherical equivalent of –1.75 to –13.25 D. One year after surgery, 76% of eyes were within 1 D of emmetropia, and 86% of eyes had unaided visual acuity of 20/40 or better. The percentage of eyes having 20/20 unaided acuity was not reported. Reoperations were done on 77% of eyes 3 or more months after the original ALK.

Comparing ALK and PRK, Mauger (1994) made the point that ALK is a riskier procedure than PRK and should be used only when other procedures are inadequate. Manche and Maloney (1997) reported complications, including symptoms of glare and halos at night, which tend to fade with time but may persist indefinitely for some patients, and problems due to the surgical procedure, including epithelial ingrowth into the interface, the presence of debris in the interface, loss of the corneal cap, and inadvertent entry into the anterior chamber. Buzard et al. (1996) commented that one deterrent to performing ALK has been the relatively high incidence of complications, primarily loss of best-corrected visual acuity resulting from induced irregular astigmatism.

In evaluating ALK, Neumann and Gulani (1997) concluded that "[a]lthough ALK has been a helpful procedure in the ongoing evolution of refractive surgery, its usefulness is being overshadowed today by LASIK. The excimer laser, capable of removing 0.25 μm of stromal tissue with each pulse, is even more accurate than even the best ALK blade."

Laser in situ Keratomileusis

LASIK, also known as "flap and zap," begins with the use of the microkeratome to remove a corneal flap as in ALK, after which the excimer laser—having been programmed for the desired correction—is used to ablate the cornea, and the superficial flap is replaced on the cornea. As with ALK, healing takes place without the use of sutures. According to Price (1995), the day after surgery the cornea is so clear that no evidence of the surgery can be seen. LASIK requires the use of a device, so FDA approval is necessary. At the time of this writing, the only available results are those from studies carried out in other countries and premarket approval studies in this country.

Pallikaris and Siganos (1997) reported on their early experience with LASIK at the University of Crete, supplying data on 43 eyes of 43 patients having preoperative refractive errors from –8.50 to –25.87 D. Intended corrections ranged from 8.00 to 16.00 D (note that a 16.00 D correction would result in a residual refractive error of –9.87 D for the most highly myopic eye). Of the 43 eyes, four developed complications and were not included in the data analysis. Two years after surgery, approximately 80% of eyes were within 2.00 D of the intended correction. Data concerning uncorrected visual acuity and loss of best-corrected acuity were not reported.

Slade et al. (1997) reported that the largest clinical study of LASIK was that of Ruiz et al. in Bogota, Colombia. The study involved 88 patients (ages not reported); 130 eyes were evaluated on all scheduled visits for a period of 1 year. Mean preoperative spherical refractive error was –3.61 D (range, –0.25 to –18.25 D), and mean cylinder error was 1.15 D (range, 0–8 D). One year after surgery, 63% of eyes were within 0.25 D of the expected correction, and uncorrected visual acuity was 20/20 or better for 67% of eyes. No patients lost two or more lines of best-corrected visual acuity. One patient required reoperation (both eyes) due to undercorrection.

In Table 10.1 (page 190), the 1-year results of this study are compared with those of the PERK study of RK and the Summit Technology study of PRK. Perhaps the most striking difference between the studies is the preoperative refractive error—as high as –18.25 D in the LASIK study, compared with –7.50 D in the PRK study. In spite of this difference, 1 year after surgery, 98% of the LASIK eyes were within ±1.00 D of the intended correction, compared with 77% of the PRK eyes, and the percentages of eyes having 20/20 acuity were virtually identical for the two studies.

In the Pallikaris and Siganos (1997) study, four eyes were excluded from the data analysis because of the following complications: anterior chamber perforation and keratoconus, intrastromal epithelial cells, macular lacquer cracks, and transient endothelial decompensation. Johnson (1997) discussed the complications of LASIK surgery, commenting that proponents of the procedure admit that complications of LASIK may be more serious than those of PRK. Decentration is a more frequent occurrence in LASIK than in PRK; haze "is still an issue and can occur with LASIK"; and irregular astigmatism is "a very serious and not infrequent problem" with LASIK.

In discussing problems with LASIK surgery, Machet (1997a), director of the Laser Center in Toronto, commented that "[j]ust as the good can be very good, the bad can be very bad." He commented that the "greatest fear" is forgetting to put the depth plate in the instrument and having the instrument automatically cut a 900-μm hole in a 550-μm cornea. In another article, Machet (1997b) explained that because the eye is under high pressure, when corneal perforation occurs "the crystalline lens is classically ejected with a burst of aqueous fluid; however, all ocular contents may be potentially lost and the corneal cap amputated."

☼ CLINICAL PEARL

As with ALK, LASIK surgery has the advantage of correcting preoperative myopia greater than –6.00 D and does not interfere with the epithelium and Bowman's membrane. As with ALK, complications of LASIK, when they occur, tend to be severe. Vision care practitioners should be aware of the amount of experience of LASIK surgeons in their locality. Nobody wants to be a surgeon's first (or even fifty-first) LASIK patient!

Intrastromal Corneal Ring

The raison d'être for the ICR is that it flattens the cornea without surgical intervention of the central cornea. A polymethyl methacrylate (PMMA) split ring is inserted into a surgically created channel in the midperiphery of the cornea. As described by Schanzlin and Verity (1997), ring thicknesses vary from 0.25 to 0.45 mm, in 0.05-mm steps, to address a range of refractive errors from approximately –1 to –6 D.

As this book goes to press, very few studies of the use of the ICR have been reported. Schanzlin and Verity (1997) have reported the results of two preliminary studies. In Sao Paulo, Brazil, 10 patients with preoperative refractive errors from –2.63 to –4.25 D underwent implantation with a 0.3-mm-thick ICR. One year after surgery, the mean reduction in spherical equivalent myopia was –2.25 ± 0.54 D. The percentages of patients within 1.00 D of emmetropia was not reported, nor was the percentage of patients with 20/20 uncorrected visual acuity. All patients were reported to have uncorrected acuity of 20/40 or better and to have best-corrected visual acuity of 20/20.

In the other study reported by Schanzlin and Verity (1997), 90 patients with refractive errors from –1.00 to –6.75 D underwent ICR implantation (in one eye only) in a phase II clinical trial. Six months after surgery, data for 63 patients indicated that 73% of eyes were within 1 D of the intended correction; 40% of eyes had uncorrected acuity of 20/20 or better; and no eyes lost two or more lines of best-corrected visual acuity. The authors concluded that "the ICR appears to be well tolerated by this group of patients, with a stable induced keratorefractive effect."

Nonthreatening complications mentioned by Schanzlin and Verity (1997) included a mild midperipheral corneal haze in the area of the stromal dissection that diminished rapidly, minute deposits within the area of the stromal channel, and the development of a superficial line of iron deposits concentric with the inner circumference of the ICR device. A more serious complication was a minute tear in Descemet's membrane, occurring in the eye of a patient in the Brazil study, that caused persistent focal edema and poor visual acuity. The problem was solved by explantation of the ring. Schanzlin and Verity commented that "the shortcoming of this form or keratorefractive surgery is that the range of correction is presently limited to low and moderate amounts of myopia."

☼ CLINICAL PEARL

In advising patients concerning keratorefractive surgery, whether RK, PRK, ALK, LASIK, or ICR, the patient should be made to understand that there is a high probability that he or she will have poorer vision—even if glasses or contact lenses are worn—than he or she had with correction before the surgery was done.

Comanagement of Refractive Surgery Patients

Because RK surgery has been an established surgical procedure for many years—with the result that many RK surgeons have already switched to the newer forms of refractive surgery—opportunities for comanagement of refractive surgery patients in the immediate future will be concerned mainly with PRK and LASIK surgery. Because engaging in these procedures requires the surgeon (or group of surgeons) to invest heavily in equipment and in its annual maintenance, refractive surgeons will need to attract a very large patient base. In view of the fact that general ophthalmologists build their practices by caring for people who have eye diseases, whereas optometrists build their practices by caring for people who have healthy ametropic eyes, the burden of supplying patients for refractive surgery will fall, to a great extent, on those optometrists who care to comanage refractive surgery patients.

Photorefractive Keratectomy Comanagement

Speaking at the Summit Technology seminar, Medina (1994) suggested that refractive surgery should be considered as an expansion of the practice of optometry and that optometrists are in a good position to comanage refractive surgery patients because 80% of the complications of refractive surgery are optical complications. He described the roles and responsibilities of the optometrist and the refractive surgeon as follows: The optometrist provides the primary care examination and consultation concerning patient expectations. The optometrist also provides preoperative evaluation, postoperative evaluation, and continued primary care. The refractive surgeon provides consultation concerning patient expectations, risks, benefits, alternative procedures, informed consent and the decision; the surgical procedure; and the postoperative evaluation. In selecting a refractive surgeon, Medina suggested that the optometrist should look for competence, experience, and interpersonal skills and that the "refracting" refractive surgeon and the "dispensing" refractive surgeon should be avoided. He also suggested that the optometrist should build his or her patient care skills, build case presentation skills, observe a range of procedures performed by a range of surgeons, and observe a range of patients in the follow-up period.

At the same seminar, Thompson (1994) discussed patient selection for PRK surgery in more detail. Medical contraindications for PRK surgery listed by Thompson included allergies, adverse reactions to medications, collagen vascular disease, pregnancy, systemic herpes zoster (which may reactivate after surgery), high IOP (because of the need for postoperative steroids), and diabetes, if unstable or with active retinopathy. As for ocular history, the patient must be at least 21 years old and must have a stable refractive error over a 3-month period. Thompson suggested that contact lens failures are good candidates, but patients having keratoconus are excluded.

Laser in situ Keratomileusis Comanagement

Making the point that many refractive surgeons have turned to LASIK surgery as their keratorefractive procedure of choice, Karpecki et al. (1997) suggested that optometrists should be knowledgeable concerning LASIK, so that when patients ask about laser vision correction they can be ready with informed and unbiased answers. Knowledge about LASIK is also important in providing preoperative and postoperative care. They made the point that LASIK can effectively correct up to approximately 12–14 D of myopia, and that current software is approved to correct up to 4.00 D of astigmatism.

Concerning complications after LASIK surgery, Karpecki et al. (1997) stated that most LASIK complications have to do with the flap. The most serious of these complications is corneal perforation, due to a missing depth plate, which is catastrophic but is unlikely to occur because new instrument designs have "all but eliminated this potential human error." A much more benign complication is an epithelial defect, requiring a bandage contact lens and a topical antibiotic-steroid combination drug. Other complications are a free corneal cap, which can be easily replaced; an incomplete cap, which requires the surgeon to postpone the laser portion of the surgery until the cornea heals; a lost cap, which requires aggressive medical therapy; and debris under the cap, which can be removed by irrigation.

How Many Photorefractive Keratectomy and Laser in situ Keratomileusis Patients Are There?

Those who encourage optometrists to comanage refractive surgery patients sometimes create the impression that optometrists who forgo this opportunity will be left with very few myopes desiring glasses or contact lenses. Is this true? Will so many myopes opt for refractive surgery that optometrists who don't engage in comanagement will be left with very little to do?

In an article titled "Has PRK's time come and gone?" O'Connor (1987) commented that although 340 laser centers had opened in the United States by the end of 1996, most struggled financially as patient demand turned out to be much less than analysts and investors anticipated. Instead of the 500,000 laser procedures expected in the United States during 1996, only about 100,000 were performed. He cited the case of Global Vision, of Jacksonville, Florida, which attracted approximately 250 optometrists to invest between $5,000 and $15,000 to become limited partners, but failed, having to close its five laser centers after losing $6 million in 2 years. He quoted Dr. Lou Catania, vice president of Global Vision, as saying, "Global spent $8,000 on radio and TV ads for every patient who paid for the $2,000 procedure."

In an article in the AOA News (July 14, 1997), Kenneth Taylor, O.D., of Arthur D. Little, Inc., was quoted as saying that even though there are 77 million myopes in the United States, the patient base for which PRK surgery is appropriate is probably only 10–12 million. This is because the FDA presently limits PRK to low to moderate myopes, in addition to excluding teens and also middle-aged persons who are about to experience presbyopia. Economics dictates that only families with annual incomes of $35,000 or more will be able to afford the procedure. Of the 10–12 million myopes, Taylor estimated that approximately 2% of the potential patient base may actually opt for PRK surgery each year.

On the basis of a survey conducted by Spectrum Consultants, reported in the AOA News (September 29, 1977), the number of laser procedures performed in the United States was projected to increase to approximately 200,000—including both PRK and LASIK procedures—during 1997. In the same issue of the AOA News, Bond-Henrickson, spokesman for Sight Resources, which operates 10 laser centers, was quoted as saying, "The most optimistic projection ever generated on the laser patient base only indicated that perhaps 0.7 percent of all vision-corrected patients would undergo the procedure." And we should not forget that when they become presbyopic, this 0.7 percent of patients will all need glasses or contact lenses.

☼ CLINICAL PEARL

Even if an optometrist chooses not to comanage refractive surgery patients, he or she should be sufficiently familiar with these procedures, including their possible unintended consequences, to be able to intelligently counsel patients, and whether or not the optometrist comanages refractive surgery patients, he or she should be competent to care for postsurgical patients who will eventually require glasses or contact lenses. Finally, it is not likely that so many myopes will opt for keratorefractive surgery that optometrists will have little or nothing to do.

References

Barr J. Optometric management of the excimer PRK patient. Seminar sponsored by Summit Technology and The Ohio State University College of Optometry. Chicago, August 1994.

Ben-Sira A, Lowenstein A, Lipshitz I, et al. Patient satisfaction after 5.0-mm photorefractive keratectomy for myopia. J Refract Surg 1997;13:128–134.

Black H. Low contrast tests may more accurately determine visual acuity post-PRK. Ocular Surg News 1997.

Bourque LG, Lynn MJ, Warning GO, Cartwright C. Spectacle and contact lens wearing six years after radial keratotomy in the prospective evaluation of radial keratotomy study. Ophthalmology 1994;101:421–431.

Brancato R, Tavola A, Corones F, et al. Excimer laser photorefractive keratectomy for myopia: results in 1165 eyes. Refract Corneal Surg 1993;9:95–194.

Bullimore ME, Sheedy JE, Owen D, Refractive Surgery Study Group. Diurnal visual changes in radial keratotomy: implications for visual standards. Optom Vis Sci 1994;71:516–521.

Buzard KA, Fundingsland BR, Friedlander M. Automated keratomileusis in situ: clinical study of 142 eyes. J Cataract Refract Surg 1996;22:1189–1199.

Casebeer JC. Comprehensive Refractive Surgery. In R Elander, LF Rich, JB Robin (eds), Principles and Practice of Refractive Surgery. Philadelphia: Saunders, 1997;8–28.

Chatterjee A, Shah S, Bessant DA, et al. Reduction in intraocular pressure after excimer laser photorefractive keratectomy. Ophthalmology 1997;104:355–359.

Dello Russo J. Is PRK the sneak thief of sight? Ocular Surg News 1997;July 15: 42–43.

Dietz MR, Sanders DR, Raanan MG, DeLuca M. Study Group. Results of the Prospective Evaluation of Radial Keratotomy (PERK) study 10 years after surgery. Arch Ophthalmol 1994;112:1298–1308.

Ditzen K, Anaschhutz T, Schroder E. Photorefractive keratectomy to treat low, medium and high myopia: a multicenter study. J Cataract Refract Surg 1994; 20(Suppl):234–238.

Duling K, Wick B. Binocular vision complications after radial keratotomy. Am J Optom Physiol Opt 1988;65:214–223.

Epstein D, Fagerholm P, Hamberg-Nystrom H, Tengroth B. Twenty-four month follow-up of excimer laser photorefractive keratectomy for myopia, refractive and visual acuity results. Ophthalmology 1994;101:1558–1564.

Forstot SL, Damiano DE. Trauma after radial keratotomy. Ophthalmology 1988;95:833–835.

Fyodorov SN, Durnev VV. Operation of dosaged dissection of corneal circular ligament in cases of myopia of mild degree. Ann Ophthalmol 1979;12:1885–1890.

Gartry S, Kerr Muir MG, Marshall J. Excimer laser photorefractive keratectomy— 18-month follow-up. Ophthalmology 1992;99:1209–1219.

Gimbel HV, Vab Westebbrygge JA, Johnson WH, et al. Visual, refractive and patient satisfaction results following bilateral photorefractive keratectomy for myopia. Refract Corneal Surg 1993;9(Suppl):5–10.

Johnson DG. Total transepithelial multipass multizone photorefractive keratectomy for myopia and astigmatism. Ocular Surg News 1997;Feb 1(Suppl):26–27.

Johnson DG. Laser in situ Keratomileusis (LASIK) Complications. In R Elander, LF Rich, JB Robin (eds), Principles and Practice of Refractive Surgery. Philadelphia: Saunders, 1997;367–370.

Karpecki PM, Uhl JG, Smith BJ, Durrie DS. How to comanage the LASIK patient. Rev Optom 1997;134:92–99.

Kim JH, Hahn TW, Lee JC, Sah WJ. Excimer laser photorefractive keratectomy for myopia: two-year follow-up. J Cataract Refract Surg 1994;20(Suppl):229–233.

L'Esperance FA, Warner JW, Telfair WB, et al. Excimer laser instrumentation and technique for human corneal surgery. Arch Ophthalmol 1989;47:131–139.

Lindstrom RL. Minimally invasive radial keratotomy: mini-RK. J Cataract Refract Surg 1997;21:27–34.

Lindstrom RL. The Barraquer Lecture: surgical management of myopia—a clinician's perspective. J Refract Surg 1997;13:287–294.

Lohman C, Gartry K, Kerr Muir M. Haze in photorefractive keratectomy: its origins and consequences. Laser Light Ophthalmol 1991;4:1534.

Lyle AW, Jin GJC. Initial results of automated lamellar keratoplasty for correction of myopia: one year follow-up. J Cataract Refract Surg 1996;22:31–43.

Machet JJ. LASIK overview: the good, the bad, and the ugly. Ocular Surg News 1997a; (Suppl):38–39.

Machet JJ. Learn the LASIK fundamentals. Ocular Surg News 1997b;March 15: 18–25.

Maguen E, Salz JJ, Nesburn AB, et al. Results of excimer laser photorefractive keratectomy for the correction of myopia. Ophthalmology 1994;101:1448–1457.

Maguire LJ. Editorial: keratorefractive surgery, success, and the public health. Am J Ophthalmol 1994;117:394–398.

Manche EF, Maloney RK. Keratomileusis for high myopia. J Cataract Refract Surg 1996;22:1443–1450.

Manche EF, Maloney RK. Myopic Keratomileusis in situ. In R Elander, LF Rich, JB Robin (eds), Principles and Practice of Refractive Surgery. Philadelphia: Saunders, 1997;227–287.

Mandelbaum S, Waring GO, Forster RK, et al. Late development of ulcerative keratitis associated with radial keratotomy scars. Arch Ophthalmol 1986;104:1156–1160.

Marshall J. The potential of lasers in refractive surgery. Trans Br Contact Lens Assoc 1989;11:63–67.

Marshall J. Optometric management of the excimer PRK patient. Seminar sponsored by Summit Technology and The Ohio State University College of Optometry. Chicago, August 1994.

Mauger T. Optometric management of the excimer PRK patient. Seminar sponsored by Summit Technology and The Ohio State University College of Optometry. Chicago, August 1994.

McDonnel PJ. Myopic photorefractive keratectomy using scanning spot (photopolishing) technique: Phase 2 results with LaserSight excimer laser. Ocular Surg News 1997;(Suppl):41–42.

Medina A. Optometric management of the excimer PRK patient. Seminar sponsored by Summit Technology and The Ohio State University College of Optometry. Chicago, August 1994.

Neumann AC, Gulani AC. Lamellar Surgeries: Counterpoint and Complications. In R Elander, LF Rich, JB Robin (eds), Principles and Practice of Refractive Surgery. Philadelphia: Saunders, 1997;291–298.

O'Connor D. Has PRK's time come and gone? Rev Optom 1987;134:76–78.

Pallikaris IG, Siganos DS. Laser in situ keratomileusis to treat myopia: early experience. J Cataract Refract Surg 1997;23:39–49.

Price FW. Update on Refractive Surgery. Lecture given at Indiana University School of Optometry. Bloomington, IN, January 1995.

Rejpal R. Optometric management of the excimer PRK patient. Seminar sponsored by Summit Technology and The Ohio State University College of Optometry. Chicago, August 1994.

Sato Y, Akiyama A, Shibata H. A new surgical approach to myopia. Am J Ophthalmol 1953;36:823–829.

Schanzlin DJ, Verity SM. Intrastromal Corneal Ring. In R Elander, LF Rich, JB Robin (eds), Principles and Practice of Refractive Surgery. Philadelphia: Saunders, 1997;415–420.

Schanzlin DJ, Santos VR, Waring GO, et al. Diurnal change in refraction, corneal curvature, visual acuity, and intraocular pressure after radial keratotomy in the PERK study. Ophthalmology 1986;93:167–175.

Seiler T, Holschbauchm A, Derse M, et al. Complications of myopic photorefractive keratectomy with the excimer laser. Ophthalmol 1994;101:144–160.

Shivitz IA, Arrowsmith PN. Delayed keratitis after radial keratotomy. Arch Ophthalmol 1986;104:1153–1155.

Simmons KG, Linsalata RP, Zaragosa AM. Ruptured globe secondary to blunt trauma following radial keratotomy. J Refract Surg 1988;4:132–135.

Slade SG, Doane JF, Ruiz LA. Laser Myopic Keratomileusis. In R Elander, LF Rich, JB Robin (eds), Principles and Practice of Refractive Surgery. Philadelphia: Saunders, 1997;357–366.

Sposato P. Report from the Institute of Contact Lens Research. Contact Lens Spectrum 1987;2:58–69.

Thompson V. Optometric management of the excimer PRK patient. Seminar sponsored by Summit Technology and The Ohio State University College of Optometry. Chicago, August 1994.

Vinger EF. Why I don't do radial keratotomy. J Am Optom Assoc 1996;67:68–72.

Waring GO. Making sense of "Keratospeak." A classification of refractive corneal surgery. Arch Ophthalmol 1985;103:1472–1477.

Waring GO, Lynn MJ, Culbertson W, et al. Three year results of the Prospective Study of Radial Keratotomy (PERK) study. Ophthalmology 1987;94:1339–1353.

Waring GO, Lynn MJ, McDonnell PJ. Results of the Prospective Evaluation of Radial Keratotomy (PERK) study 10 years after surgery. Arch Ophthalmol 1994;112:1298–1308.

Waring GO, Lynn MJ, Gelender H, et al. Results of the Prospective Evaluation of Radial Keratotomy (PERK) study one year after surgery. Ophthalmology 1985;92:177–208.

CHAPTER 11

Refractive Surgery Involving the Lens

If today the only means available for correcting myopia consisted of [surgery] and tomorrow somebody invented glasses or contacts, he'd win the Nobel Prize hands down.

"Myopic Haste," *Forbes Magazine*, May 6, 1985

Clear Lens Extraction

Clear lens extraction followed by implantation of an intraocular lens (IOL) has been a controversial form of myopia correction because of the possibility of retinal detachment associated with this procedure. Not only is the risk of retinal detachment in undisturbed phakic eyes much greater for myopic eyes than for emmetropic or hyperopic eyes—for example, Perkins (1979) estimated that the risk of retinal detachment is 330 times greater in eyes having refractive errors above –10.00 D than in eyes having refractive errors between plano and +4.75 D—but also lens removal and IOL implantation, are accompanied by a risk of retinal detachment. For a young myope, there is the additional problem of loss of the ability to accommodate.

Among the more recent reports of clear lens extraction are those of Barraquer et al. (1994) in Bogota, Colombia; Colin and Robinet (1994) in Brest, France; Gris et al. (1996) in Barcelona, Spain; and Lee and Lee (1996) in Seoul, Korea. Barraquer et al. (1994) reported retrospective data on 165 eyes of 107 pathologic myopes who underwent clear lens extraction between 1980 and 1990. Mean preoperative myopia was –21.50 ± 6.65 D, and mean age was 34 ± 15 years. The authors provided no information concerning postoperative visual acuity, uncorrected or corrected, and no information concerning the method of correction (spectacles or contact lenses) for the 156 eyes that were not implanted with an IOL.

Colin and Robinet (1994) reported the results of clear lens extraction and implantation of posterior chamber IOLs in 52 eyes of 30 patients 22–51 years of age, with 1-year follow-up. Preoperative spherical equivalent refractive errors ranged from –12.00 to –23.75 D. Prophylactic argon laser photocoagulation was performed for 31 eyes that had lattice degeneration or a focal tear or hole. One year postoperatively 64% of eyes were within 1.00 D of emmetropia. Corrected visual acuity was 20/20 or better for two eyes before surgery and four eyes after surgery and was 20/40 or better for 37 eyes before surgery and 42 eyes (89%) after surgery.

Gris et al. (1996) reviewed the results of clear lens extraction for 46 eyes of 37 patients. Ages ranged from 29 to 56 years, with a mean of 38 years, and mean preoperative spherical equivalent refractive error was –16.05 ± 5.01 D. Polymethyl methacrylate (PMMA) IOLs were implanted in the lens capsule in all but two eyes, in which they were implanted in the ciliary sulcus. The mean IOL power was +6.67 D: No negative IOLs were implanted, but zero-power IOLs were implanted in 17 eyes (40%). Postoperatively, 48% of eyes were within 1 D of emmetropia, and 93% were within 2 D. No information was given concerning unaided visual acuity postoperatively, but the authors stated that best-corrected visual acuity was 20/40 or better in 69% of eyes before surgery and in 89% of eyes after surgery and that the surgery did not impair best-corrected acuity in any eye.

Lee and Lee (1996) reported retrospective data on 24 eyes of 16 patients whose ages ranged from 22 to 52 years with a mean of 34 years. The mean preoperative refractive error was –16.60 D, with a range from –12.00 to –25.75 D. Targeted postoperative refractive errors ranged from emmetropia to –3.00 D for 20 patients, but for four patients targeted refractive errors were from +0.60 to +1.40 D because of the unavailability of low-power plus IOLs. Postoperatively, 63% of eyes were within 1.00 D of the targeted refractive error and 96% of eyes were with 2.00 D, with 38% of eyes having unaided acuity of 20/40 or better. No information was given concerning the number of eyes (if any) having unaided acuity of 20/20. Best-corrected acuity improved after surgery in 86% of eyes, and there were no eyes for which best-corrected acuity decreased after surgery.

A graph published by Lee and Lee (1996) indicated that preoperative best-corrected acuity was 20/100 or worse for three eyes, from 20/32 to 20/50 for six eyes, and from 20/30 to 20/20 for the remaining 15 eyes. Although not mentioned by the authors, this relatively poor best-corrected preoperative acuity—coupled with the fact that improvement occurred postoperatively for all but 4 of the eyes—must have been at least partially due to the greatly increased retinal image size that occurs when a highly myopic eye is corrected with a lens within the eye as compared with a spectacle lens at some distance in front of the eye. It is also possible that subclinical lens opacities may have contributed to the poor preoperative acuity (the authors' exclusion criteria apparently did not include lens opacities).

Complications

In their retrospective study of 165 eyes, Barraquer et al. (1994) reported the following complications:

1. Fifty-six eyes developed a secondary opacity of the posterior capsule, at an average time of 25.6 months after lens extraction. The opacities were treated with surgical discission for 11 eyes and with Nd:YAG (neodymium:yttrium-aluminum-garnet) laser surgery for 45 eyes.
2. Retinal detachment occurred in 12 eyes (7.3%), in six of which Nd:YAG laser capsulotomy had been performed. The detachments occurred 1.5–66.0 months after surgery. No information was given concerning visual acuity after reattachment surgery.

Complications reported by Colin and Robinet (1994) in their series of 52 eyes included

1. Subfoveal choroidal neovascularization that occurred in one eye 9 months after surgery, which caused acuity to decrease from 20/50 to 20/200
2. Posterior capsular opacification, requiring Nd:YAG laser capsulotomy, that occurred in four eyes
3. Posterior vitreous detachment in 30 eyes

The authors reported that there were no cases of cystoid macular edema, retinal detachment, or persistent corneal edema. They concluded that the lack of retinal detachments could be attributed to the prophylactic argon laser photocoagulation performed for 31 eyes that had lattice degeneration, tears, or holes.

Complications reported by Gris et al. (1996) included the following:

1. A posterior capsule tear with vitreous loss occurred in one eye.
2. A capsule break without a tear occurred in one eye.
3. Four weeks after surgery, retinal detachment occurred in the eye with the capsular tear. After surgical repair, visual acuity was 20/20.
4. A post-traumatic iris collapse occurred in one eye.
5. A subclinical IOL decentration occurred in one eye.
6. Significant posterior capsular opacities occurred in three eyes, at 4, 7, and 13 months. In each of these three eyes, Nd:YAG laser posterior capsulotomy was performed.

In spite of these complications, Gris et al. concluded that clear lens extraction is an effective, inexpensive, and safe procedure for correcting myopia in middle-aged patients, but they commented that many authors consider it to be a high-risk procedure for younger patients.

The only complication reported by Lee and Lee (1996) during a 12- to 20-month follow-up period was posterior capsule opacification, occurring

4 months postoperatively in one eye. Successful Nd:YAG laser posterior capsulotomy was performed. They commented, however, that retinal detachment may occur years after the surgery. Lee and Lee concluded that clear lens extraction is effective in reducing severe myopia, but the safety of the procedure should be evaluated with longer follow-up of larger numbers of cases.

Werblin (1997) discussed a study by Centurian et al. (submitted for publication) of 35 highly myopic patients who were followed for 7 years after clear lens extraction. There was no incidence of retinal detachment during the 7-year period. Werblin attributed the lack of retinal detachments to the fact that all eyes underwent prophylactic argon laser photocoagulation before surgery, with focal treatment for all lesions, including lattice degeneration, holes, and tears. Werblin commented that using the reported rates (0.7% per year) for detachment for unoperated eyes fitting the criteria for those in the study, between one and two detachments would have been expected for the 35 subjects if the surgery had not been done. He discussed new approaches in surgical procedures and IOL design, and concluded that higher degrees of refractive accuracy are theoretically possible and "[t]hus the potential exists for a safe, accurate, stable surgical modality whose risk-benefit ratio is comparable to that of contact lenses or glasses."

The results of the studies of clear lens extraction are summarized in Table 11.1.

Critiques of Clear Lens Extraction

In a critical review of the literature on clear lens extraction, Goldberg (1987), a retinal surgeon at the University of Illinois, tabulated data from several studies showing that the incidence of retinal detachment after lens extraction varies from 0 to 0.9% in nonmyopic eyes but from 3.5% to 9.5% in myopic eyes. He also tabulated data from several studies concerning visual acuity after reattachment surgery, showing that percentages of eyes having visual acuity of 20/50 or worse vary from 48% to 77%. After discussing other possible complications of lens extraction—including opacification of the posterior capsule and cystoid macular edema—Goldberg made the following comments:

> The time-honored physician's principle of *primum non nocere* is reinforced by the availability of alternatives (including nonsurgical refractive devices) that are safer than clear lens extraction. Based on the available evidence, therefore, I conclude that the risk/benefit ratio for this operation is currently too high for it to be recommended.

In a more recent critique of clear lens extraction, Kaufman and Kaufman (1997) referred to Goldberg's critical review (with which, in general, they

TABLE 11.1
Results of Studies of Clear Lens Extraction and Replacement
with an Intraocular Lens

	Barraquer et al. (1994)	*Colin and Robinet (1996)*	*Gris et al. (1996)*	*Lee and Lee (1996)*
Number of eyes	165	52	46	24
Ages of subjects (yrs)	34 ± 15	22–51	29–56	22–52
Initial refractive error (D)	–21.5 ± 6.7	–12 to –23.7	–16.1 ± 5.1	–12.0 to –25.8
Residual refractive error (within ±1.00 D)	Not reported	64%	48%	63%
Uncorrected acuity (20/20 or better)	Not reported	38%	Not reported	38%

agreed), saying that the procedure is "technically simple but may be accompanied by various complications. . . . the complication rate associated with this procedure may be markedly higher than that of phakic IOL implantation procedures."

☀ CLINICAL PEARL

Obvious advantages of clear lens extraction are that it does not affect the optical quality of the cornea and that very large amounts of myopia can be reduced or eliminated. However, the possibility that retinal detachment can occur—even months or years after surgery—makes this a questionable procedure. It is probable that many years will have to elapse before it is known whether improvements in surgical procedures and IOL implantation will someday reduce the risk of retinal detachment and other complications to near-zero levels.

Intraocular Lens Implantation in a Phakic Eye

In young patients, accommodation can be preserved by implanting an IOL in the anterior or posterior chamber without extracting the crystalline lens. At a symposium on cataract and refractive surgery, Waring (reported by DuBosar, 1997) noted that anterior chamber lenses for myopia were first used in Europe in the 1950s, along with anterior chamber lenses for aphakia. These thick, vaulted lenses resulted in complications, including endothelial cell loss, corneal edema, hyphema, uveitis, and glaucoma, with the result that approximately half of the lenses implanted were eventually explanted. In 1987, Fyodorov and colleagues in Russia first reported on implantation of posterior chamber lenses in phakic myopic eyes (Fechner et al., 1996).

Anterior Chamber Lenses

Baikoff (1997) reported on a study conducted in France, beginning in 1990, for the purpose of observing endothelial changes occurring after the anterior chamber lens implantation. Each of nine surgical centers implanted 15 patients with the Chiron Domilens (Chiron Vision, Claremont, CA). The patients ranged in age from 25 to 45 years and had myopia ranging from –7 to –25 D. For each patient, one eye was initially operated, and if the second eye was to be operated, this was done 6 months later. Implant powers ranged from –8 to –15 D. Twenty-three patients who required implants stronger than –15 D were deliberately undercorrected. At the time of Baikoff's report, follow-up data were available for periods varying from 1 to 3 years. Mean uncorrected visual acuity was 20/40, and mean corrected acuity was 20/30. Residual refractive errors were relatively stable during the 3-year period, with 50–65% of eyes having a refractive error within 1 D of emmetropia.

The research team decided that the study would be discontinued if endothelial cell loss was greater than 15%. Graphs published by Baikoff (1997) showed that endothelial cell loss increased only slightly during the 3-year period. At 3 years, mean endothelial cell loss was 5.5 ± 9% in the central cornea and 3.9 ± 10% in the peripheral cornea: These losses were found not to be statistically significant.

Pérez-Santonja et al. (1997) conducted a study in which the Worst-Fechner iris fixated anterior chamber lens (Ophtec BV, Grohingen, The Netherlands) was implanted in 32 phakic eyes of 19 patients having myopia ranging from –9.50 to –27.00 D. Postoperative tests, in addition to refractive error and visual acuity measurement, included measurement of endothelial cell density by means of specular microscopy, measurement of lens transmittance (for 20 eyes) by means of fluorophotometry, and monitoring of anterior chamber inflammation (for 30 eyes) using a laser flare cell photometer. Because IOLs were not available in the powers needed to achieve emmetropia for many of the eyes, a full correction was attempted for only 24 of the 32 eyes. The mean refractive error at 3 months postoperatively for these 24 eyes was +0.28 D, and the mean refractive error for 11 of the 24 eyes refracted 2 years postoperatively was –0.08 D. Visual acuity data showed that for 17 eyes on which acuity was measured at 2 years, mean uncorrected visual acuity was 20/44, and mean spectacle-corrected visual acuity was 20/33. Endothelial cell loss was 7.2% at 3 months and 17.6% at 2 years postoperatively; loss in lens transmittance was 0.62% at 3 months and 1.03% at 18 months; and postoperative flare results indicated a chronic subclinical inflammation between 1 and 2 years after implantation.

The results of the studies of anterior chamber IOL implantation in phakic eyes are summarized in Table 11.2.

TABLE 11.2
Results of Studies of Anterior Chamber Lens Implantation in Phakic Eyes

	Baikoff (1997)	*Perez-Santonja et al. (1997)*
Number of eyes	135	32
Ages of subjects (yrs)	25–45	≥20
Initial refractive error (D)	–7.0 to –25.0	–9.5 to –27.0
Residual refractive error		
Within ±1.00 D	50–65%	
Mean		+0.28 D*
Uncorrected acuity (mean)	20/40	20/44

*Three-month data on 24 eyes for which lenses of the desired power were available.

Complications

Baikoff (1997) reported the following complications with the Chiron Domilens:

1. Retinal detachment occurred in one eye, 2 years after surgery, on lattice degeneration sights that had previously been photocoagulated. The retina was reattached "without anatomic or functional complications to the eye."
2. Early uveitis occurred in three eyes, one of which had preexisting ocular hypertension, and explantation was done on the second postoperative day. The other two eyes responded to medical treatment.
3. Uveitis occurred in one eye at 3 months, which responded to medical therapy.
4. Rotation or displacement of the implant occurred in nine eyes. In these eyes, the implant was either removed without being replaced, or was removed and replaced by a new implant.
5. Thirty-seven patients complained of halos, dazzling, or glare, occurring at night. Baikoff reported that "[p]atients grew tolerant of halos and glare . . . glare persisted in only 24 cases." No cases of induced cataract were reported.

Complications reported by Pérez-Santonja et al. (1997) with the Worst-Fechner lens included the following:

1. Postoperative uveitis (three eyes) that improved with corticosteroid eye drops
2. Pigment disposition on the endothelium (six eyes) occurring 6–18 months after surgery
3. Subconjunctival fistula (six eyes), requiring resuturing of the wound
4. Elevated intraocular pressure (five eyes) thought to be steroid induced

5.   IOL decentration greater than 0.25 mm (22 of the 32 eyes)
6.   Complaints of halos (18 eyes), mainly in those eyes with the larger amounts of IOL decentration
7.   An anterior subcapsular lens opacity occurred in one eye, not involving the visual axis.

Pérez-Santonja et al. concluded that a continual decrease in endothelial cell density, a decrease in lens transmittance, a chronic subclinical inflammation, decentration of the IOL, "and other potential hazards of Worst-Fechner lens implantation should restrict the application of this method to patients under controlled clinical investigation until long-term results concerning its safety are evaluated."

Posterior Chamber Lenses

Results of the implantation of silicone posterior chamber IOLs in 69 phakic eyes of 37 myopes in Hanover, Germany, were reported by Fechner et al. (1996). Mean preoperative refractive error was –16.20 D, with a range of –8.00 to –39.60 D. Ages of patients were not reported. The Chiron Adatomed lens, used for all eyes, has a posterior radius of curvature of 9.9 mm, which closely approximates the radius of the anterior surface of the crystalline lens. Three months after surgery, the deviation of the achieved refraction from the predicted refraction in 53 eyes varied from +1.77 to –2.80 D, and no eye lost best-corrected acuity. The authors provided no information concerning uncorrected visual acuity, nor did they say how they arrived at the "predicted refraction."

Also using the Chiron Adatomed posterior chamber lens, Marinho et al. (1997) implanted the lens in 38 phakic eyes of 24 consecutive patients having myopia from –7.00 to –28.00 D, with follow-up ranging from 3 to 24 months. Refractive errors 3 months after surgery were between +1.00 and –1.00 D for 27 of the 32 eyes, and 24 of the 32 eyes gained two or more lines of spectacle-corrected acuity. Unaided visual acuity after surgery was not reported.

Assetto et al. (1996) of Torino, Italy, reported on the implantation of collagen polymer IOLs in 15 phakic eyes of 14 patients with spherical equivalent refractive errors from –10.8 to –24.0 D, with a mean of –15.30 ± 3.10 D. They described the IOL, which they referred to as an "implantable contact lens," as having a concave posterior surface "which vaults over the lens capsule to provide space for the aqueous." Postoperatively, the mean spherical equivalent refraction was –2.00 ± 3.10 D; 31% of eyes had less than 1.00 D of residual myopia; and none of the eyes were hyperopic. As shown in one of their graphs, eight eyes had uncorrected acuity of 20/40 or better, one of which had uncorrected acuity of 20/20. Best-corrected visual acuity improved in all eyes but one, in which it decreased from 20/30 to 20/40.

TABLE 11.3
Results of Studies of Posterior Chamber Lens Implantation in Phakic Eyes

	Fechner et al. (1996)	Marinho et al. (1997)	Assetto et al. (1996)
Number of eyes	69	38	15
Ages of subjects (yrs)	Not reported	24	Not reported
Initial refractive error (D)	–8.0 to –39.6	–7.0 to –28.0	–10.8 to –24.0
Residual refractive error (within ±1.00 D)	Not reported	71%	31%
Uncorrected acuity (20/20)	Not reported	Not reported	7% (one eye)

The results of the studies of posterior chamber IOL implantation in phakic eyes are summarized in Table 11.3.

Complications

Fechner et al. (1996) reported the following complications of posterior chamber lens implantation:

1. In one eye, a preexisting lens opacity close to the optic axis increased in density during the first postoperative week, with the result that the IOL was removed and the cataractous lens was extracted.
2. Both eyes of one patient "reacted violently" to IOL insertion, causing crystalline lens opacities within a few days, after which the cataractous lenses were removed and replaced by posterior chamber IOLs.
3. The lenses implanted in four eyes were too small (10.5 mm in diameter), causing marked decentration, and were removed and replaced with larger IOLs.
4. Cortical opacities appeared 1–2 years postoperatively in eight of 45 eyes that had clear or almost clear cortexes preoperatively. In all of these eyes, there was no visible space between the IOL and the crystalline lens. None of these opacities impeded visual acuity, but "it appeared likely that they would in the future."

Fechner et al. concluded that "until the frequency of cataract inducement is clarified by further observation, the decision to implant this posterior chamber myopia lens should be considered carefully."

Marinho et al. (1997) reported the following complications:

1. Moderate glare was reported (six eyes).
2. Severe glare was reported in both eyes of one patient, who "demanded explantation 3 months after surgery."
3. Moderate uveitis was reported (two eyes).

4. The IOL was not correctly positioned in one eye, causing corneal touch and focal edema. The IOL was explanted and replaced by a Baikoff anterior chamber IOL.
5. A retinal detachment occurred in 9 months (one eye), which was successfully managed by a vitreoretinal surgeon.

Assetto et al. (1996) reported that (1) IOL decentration occurred in six eyes (of six patients), due to the lens being too short for ciliary sulcus fixation, causing four of the six patients to complain of glare and nocturnal diplopia, and (2) pigment deposits were seen on four lenses, which cleared in 4 weeks. Assetto et al. commented that the refractive results were not totally satisfactory but that improvements in the lens design and the power calculations should significantly reduce the need for secondary surgical intervention.

☀ CLINICAL PEARL

Although IOL implantation in a phakic eye shares the advantages of IOL implantation after clear lens extraction of not affecting the optical quality of the cornea and being able to reduce or eliminate very large amounts of myopia, many problems with this procedure still need to be addressed. As with IOL implantation after clear lens extraction, many years may have to elapse before it is known whether improvements in surgical procedures and IOL implantation will someday reduce the risk of postoperative complications to acceptable levels.

References

Assetto V, Benedetti S, Pesando P. Collamer intraocular contact lens to correct high myopia. J Cataract Refract Surg 1996;22:551–556.

Baikoff GD. Refractive Phakic Intraocular Lenses. In R Elander, LF Rich, JB Robin (eds), Principles and Practice of Refractive Surgery. Philadelphia: Saunders, 1997;435–448.

Barraquer C, Cavalier C, Mejia LF. Incidence of retinal detachment following clear lens extraction in myopic patients. Arch Ophthalmol 1994;112:336–339.

Colin J, Robinet A. Clear lensectory and implantation of low-power posterior chamber intraocular lens for the correction of high myopia. Ophthalmology 1994;101:107–112.

DuBosar R. Experts discuss history and what's new with phakic IOLs. Ocular Surg News 1997;15:45–51.

Fechner PU, Haigis W, Wichmann W. Posterior chamber myopia lenses in phakic eyes. J Cataract Refract Surg 1996;22:178–182.

Goldberg MF. Clear lens extraction for axial myopia, an appraisal. Ophthalmology 1987;94:571–582.

Gris O, Guell JJ, Manero F, Muller A. Clear lens extraction to correct high myopia. J Cataract Refract Surg 1996;22:686–689.

Kaufman SC, Kaufman HE. Phakic Intraocular Lenses and Clear Lens Extraction for High Myopia: Counterpoint. In R Elander, LF Rich, JB Robin (eds), Principles and Practice of Refractive Surgery. Philadelphia: Saunders, 1997;459–474.

Lee KH, Lee JH. Long term results of clear lens extraction for severe myopia. J Cataract Refract Surg 1996;22:1411–1415.

Marinho A, Neves MC, Pinto MC, Vaz F. Posterior chamber silicone phakic intraocular lenses. J Refract Surg 1997;13:219–222.

Pérez-Santonja JJ, Bueno JL, Zato MA. Surgical correction of high myopia in phakic eyes with Worst-Fechner myopia intraocular lenses. J Refract Surg 1997;13: 268–284.

Perkins ES. Morbidity from myopia. Sight Sav Rev 1979;49:11–19.

Werblin TF. Clear Lens/Cataract Extraction for Refractive Purposes. In R Elander, LF Rich, JB Robin (eds), Principles and Practice of Refractive Surgery. Philadelphia: Saunders, 1997;449–458.

Index

Note: Page numbers followed by *f* indicate figures;
page numbers followed by *t* indicate tables.

Accommodation
  anomalies of, 67
  comparison between lenses and spec-
    tacles, 87–88
  as factor in prescribing for myopia,
    79–84
  fatigue of, 67
  infacility of, 67
  paralysis of, 68
  spasm of, 67
Accommodative insufficiency
  as factor in prescribing for myopia, 81
  symptoms of myopia due to, 67–68
Accommodative responses, 55–57,
    56f, 57f
Added plus power, for near work, con-
    trol with, 113–127. *See also*
    Near work, added plus power
    for, control with
Adrenergic blocking agents, myopia
    control with, 133–134, 135t
Adult(s), young. *See* Young adults
Adult acceleration, 28, 29, 30f
Adult continuation, 28, 29, 29f
Adult stabilization, 28–29, 28f
Age, as factor in prescribing for myopia,
    77–78
Alternating cover test, in binocular
    vision examination, 71
Anisometropia, comparison between
    lenses and spectacles, 87

Anterior chamber lenses, in phakic eye,
    212–214, 213t
  complications of, 213–214
  studies of, 213t
Apomorphine, myopia control with,
    future possibilities with,
    135–136
Astigmatism
  comparison between lenses and spec-
    tacles, 88
  correction of, radial keratotomy in,
    185–186
Atrophy, chorioretinal, 35
Atropine
  and bifocals, studies of, 131–132
  myopia control with, 130–131
    future possibilities with, 134–135
Automated lamellar keratoplasty,
    197–198
Axial power, 146
Axial radius, 146

Baltimore project, 101–102
Behavioral training methods, studies of,
    in vision therapy, 105–107
Berkeley Orthokeratology Study,
    165–166, 166f
Bifocal(s), for near work, 113–125,
    115t–117t
  effect of phoria status on reduction of
    progression rates with, 121–125

Bifocal(s) – *continued*
  power in, 126
  prospective studies conducted in clinics, 119–121
  studies analyzing private practice patient records, 114–119, 115t–117t
Bifocal rigid gas-permeable contact lenses, myopia control with, 162–163
Binder et al. Orthokeratology Study, 165
Binocular vision, anomalies of, symptoms of myopia due to, 65–68
Binocular vision examination, 70–74
  cover tests in, 70–72
  fixation disparity tests in, 73–74
  "flash" method in, 72
  tests of dissociated phoria in, 72
  tests of fusional vergence reserves in, 73
  von Graefe dissociated phoria test in, 72
Biofeedback studies, in vision therapy, 102–105
Biomicroscopy, in ocular health examination, 75
Blurred distance vision, 63–65, 64t, 65t
  due to congenital conditions, 64

Casebeer system, in radial keratotomy, 185
Cataract(s), probability of, 40
Central fundus, pathologic changes in, 31–35
Children
  bifocals for, studies of, 113–125, 115t–117t
  prescribing for myopia in, 77–78
  prevalence of myopia among, 9–11, 10t
  progression of myopia in, 21–24
    ocular optical component changes in, 26–28, 27f, 27t
    rates of, 51, 52f
    factors affecting, 24–26, 25t, 26f
Chiron Domilens, 212–214
Chorioretinal atrophy, 35
Choroidal crescent, 31
Classification of myopia, 14–16
  congenital, 14
  early adult–onset, 15
  induced, 15

  intermediate, 16
  late adult–onset, 15
  night, 15
  pathologic, 15
  physiologic, 16
  pseudomyopia, 15
  simple, 15, 16
  youth-onset, 14–15
Clear lens extraction, 207–211
  complications of, 209–210, 211t
  controversial issues of, 207
  critiques of, 210–211
Clinical examination, 63–76
  binocular vision, 70–74
  blurred distance vision, 63–65, 64t, 65t
  ocular health, 74–76
  refractive, 68–69
Congenital myopia, 14
Contact lenses
  corneal topography changes due to, screening for, 151–152
  fitting of, after radial keratotomy, 186
  vs. glasses, 86–91
  need for, after radial keratotomy, 183
  peripheral keratometry in, 141–142, 142f
  polymethyl methacrylate, myopia control with, 156
  rigid. *See* Rigid contact lenses
  soft
    as factor in prescribing for myopia, 91
    myopia control with, 156–157
    and spectacles, optical comparison of, 87–88
Contex OK lens
  fitting of, 168–170
  lenses in, 169
Control of myopia, 155–180
  bifocal rigid gas-permeable contact lenses in, 162–163
  methods of, 58
  with polymethyl methacrylate lenses, 156
  soft contact lenses in, 156–157
Conventional orthokeratology, video-keratoscopy in, 150
Convergence excess, as factor in prescribing for myopia, 80–81

Convergence insufficiency, 66
    as factor in prescribing for myopia, 84
Corneal haze, 188–189
Corneal Modeling System, 145
Corneal topography, 139–154
    changes in, screening for, contact
        lens wear and, 151–152
    in keratoconus detection, 143, 143f
    peripheral keratometry in, 139–143,
        140f–143f
    photokeratoscopy in, 144
    postoperative monitoring in,
        152–153
    videokeratoscopy in, 144–153. *See also*
        Ocular health examination
CorneaScope, 144
Cover tests in binocular vision examina-
        tion, 70–72
    alternating, 71
    prism-neutralized, 71–72
    subjective, 71
    unilateral, 70
Crack(s), lacquer, 33
Crescent(s), optic nerve, 31–32
Cup/disk ratio, 32
Cycloplegic agents, myopia control with,
        129–133, 133t
    atropine, 130–131
        future possibilities with, 134–135
    tropicamide, 132–133, 133t

Developmental conditions, blurred dis-
        tance vision due to, 64
Dilated fundus examination, in ocular
        health examination, 75–76
Dioptric curvature maps, 147
Dissociated phoria, tests of, 72
Distance vision, blurred, 63–65, 64t, 65t
    due to congenital conditions, 64
Distance visual acuity, myopia and,
        relationship between, 63–64,
        64t, 65t
Divergence excess, 66
    as factor in prescribing for
        myopia, 83

Early adult–onset myopia, 15
Ectasia, formation of, 33, 34f
Emmetropia, refractive error of, myopia
        due to, 16–18, 17t, 18f

Emmetropization, 54
Environmental factors, myopia due to,
        49–52
    physiologic mechanisms in, 51–58
Epidemiology, 3–48
    classification, 14–16
    optics of myopic eye, 3–8
    prevalence, 8–14
    progression, 21–31
Esophoria
    nearpoint, as factor in prescribing for
        myopia, 90–91
    symptoms of myopia due to, 66
Ethical issues, radial keratotomy–related,
        186–187
Etiology, 49–62
    environmental factors, 49–58
    inheritance and, 49–58
Exophoria
    basic, as factor in prescribing for
        myopia, 83
    symptoms of myopia due to, 66
Expansion glaucoma, 40

Fatigue of accommodation, symptoms
        of myopia due to, 67
Field of view, comparison between
        lenses and spectacles, 87
Fixation disparity tests, in binocular
        vision examination, 73–74
"Flap and zap," 198–199
"Flash" method, in binocular vision
        examination, 72
Fuchs' spot, 35
Fusional vergence reserves, tests of, in
        binocular vision examina-
        tion, 73

Glare
    after radial keratotomy, 182–183
    vision in, after laser photorefractive
        keratectomy, 194–195
Glasses
    vs. contact lenses, 86–91
    need for, after radial keratotomy, 183
Glaucoma, probability of, 40
Glaucomatous cupping, 33

Haze, corneal, 188–189
Hemorrhage(s), retinal, 33

Heterophoria(s), symptoms of myopia
    due to, 65–67
Hong Kong, prevalence of myopia in, 14
Houston Orthokeratology Study,
    164–165
Houston Rigid Gas-Permeable Myopia
    Control Study, 157–162, 159f,
    160f, 161t
Hyperopia, very low, myopia due to,
    16–18, 17t, 18f
Hyperopic drift, after radial keratot-
    omy, 184

Induced myopia, 15
    as factor in prescribing for myopia,
        94–95
Induced phoria, 66
Infacility of accommodation, symptoms
    of myopia due to, 67
Inheritance, myopia due to, 49–58
Instantaneous power, 146
Instantaneous radius, 146
Intermediate myopia, 16
Intraocular lens implantation, in phakic
    eye, 211–216
    anterior chamber lenses, 212–214, 213t
    posterior chamber lenses,
        214–216, 215t
Intraocular pressure, after laser photore-
    fractive keratectomy, 196
Intrastromal corneal ring, 200

Keratectomy, laser photorefractive. *See*
    Laser photorefractive keratec-
    tomy
Keratitis, after radial keratotomy, 184
Keratoconus
    detection of, 143, 143f
    preoperative screening for, 151
Keratometry
    peripheral
        in contact lens practice,
            141–142, 142f
        in corneal topography measure-
            ment, 139–143, 140f–143f
        and videokeratoscopy, comparison
            of, 147–148, 148f
    in refractive examination, 68–69
Keratomileusis, 197–198
Keratorefractive surgery, 181–206

automated lamellar keratoplasty,
    197–198
comanagement of patients, 201–203
intrastromal corneal ring, 200
laser photorefractive keratectomy,
    187–197
LASIK, 198–199
    comanagement of patients, 202
    prevalence of, 203–204
radial keratotomy, 181–187
videokeratoscopy, 150–151
Keratoscope, Photo-Electronic, 144
Keratotomy
    mini-radial, 185
    radial, 181–187. *See also* Radial kera-
        totomy

Labetalol, myopia control with, 134, 135t
Lacquer cracks, 33
Laser in situ keratomileusis (LASIK),
    198–199
    comanagement of patients, 202
    prevalence of, 203–204
Laser photorefractive keratectomy,
    187–197
    evaluation of, 190–195, 191t, 192f, 193f
    healing process after, 188–189, 189f
    innovations in, 196–197
    intraocular pressure after, 196
    loss of best-corrected visual acuity
        after, 191–192
    myopic drift after, 192–193, 192f, 193f
    night vision problems after, 195
    procedure, 188–189, 189f
    refractive error and visual acuity
        after, 190–191, 191t
    regression of surgical effect after,
        192–193, 192f, 193f
    scanning beam excimer laser in,
        196–197
    Summit Technology Study, 189, 190t
    transepithelial photorefractive kera-
        tectomy ablation, 197
    vision in glare after, 194–195
    vision in low contrast after, 194
    visual effects of, 193–195
LASIK. *See* Laser in situ keratomileusis
    (LASIK)
Late adult–onset myopia, 15
Lattice degeneration, 36

Legal issues, radial keratotomy–related, 186–187
Lens changes, blurred distance vision due to, 65
Low contrast, vision in, after laser photorefractive keratectomy, 194

Mini-radial keratotomy, 185
Morbidity, ocular. *See* Ocular morbidity
Mountford's fitting method, 174
Myopia. *See also* Epidemiology; *specific considerations related to, e.g.,* Clinical examination
behavioral definition of, 3
control, 3
with pharmaceutical agents, 129–137. *See also* Pharmaceutical agents, myopia control with
correction, 3
near work–induced, 58
optical definition of, 3
reduction, 3
Myopic conus, 31
Myopic disk cupping, 32–33
Myopic drift, after laser photorefractive keratectomy, 192–193, 192f, 193f
Myopic eye, optics of, 3–8
comparison studies, 4–7, 6t–9t
correlation studies, 4, 5t

Nasal supertraction, 32
Near work, added plus power for, control with, 113–127
bifocals in, 113–125
myopia induced by, 58
part-time wear of spectacles, 125–126
patient education in, 126–127
progressive addition lenses, 125
undercorrection, 125
Nearpoint esophoria, as factor in prescribing for myopia, 90–91
Negative fusional vergence reserve, 73
Neovascularization, subretinal, 35
Newborn(s), prevalence of myopia among, 9, 10t
Night myopia, 15
as factor in prescribing for myopia, 92–93

Night vision problems, after laser photorefractive keratectomy, 195
Nonexpansion glaucoma, 40

Ocular health examination, 74–76
biomicroscopy in, 75
dilated fundus examination in, 75–76
direct ophthalmoscopy in, 74–75
tonometry in, 75
visual field screening in, 75
Ocular morbidity, 39–41, 40t
blind registrations, 39
cataracts, 40
glaucoma, 39–40
retinal detachment, 39, 40t
Ocular optical component changes
in children, 26–28, 27f, 27t
in young adult myopia progression, 29–31
Ophthalmoscopy, direct, in ocular health examination, 74–75
Optic(s), of myopic eye, 3–8. *See also* Myopic eye, optics of
Optic nerve crescents, 31–32
Orthofocus technique, 163
Orthokeratology
accelerated
case reports, 170–172
Mountford's fitting method in, 174
vs. refractive surgery, 175–177, 176f
results with, 170–174
retrospective and prospective studies, 172–174, 173f
with reverse geometry lenses, 167–177. *See also* Reverse geometry lenses, accelerated orthokeratology with
videokeratoscopy in, 150
videokeratoscopy in, 175
conventional, videokeratoscopy in, 150
defined, 163
after refractive surgery, 177–178
rigid contact lenses, 163–167. *See also* Rigid contact lenses, orthokeratology with

Pacific University Orthokeratology Study, 166–167, 168t
Paralysis of accommodation, symptoms of myopia due to, 68

Pathologic changes, 31–38
    case report, 38
    in central fundus, 31–35
    chorioretinal atrophy, 35
    Fuchs' spot, 35
    lacquer cracks, 33
    lattice degeneration, 36
    myopic disk cupping, 32–33
    optic nerve crescents, 31–32
    paving-stone degeneration, 36
    in peripheral fundus, 36–37
    pigmentary degeneration, 36
    posterior staphyloma formation,
        33, 34f
    retinal breaks, 36
    retinal detachment, 37–38
    retinal hemorrhages, 33
    subretinal neovascularization, 35
    vitreous detachment, 35–36, 36–37, 37f
    white-without-pressure, 36
Pathologic myopia, 15
Patient education, in near work eye
        control, 126–127
Paving-stone degeneration, 36
Peripheral keratometry
    in contact lens practice, 141–142, 142f
    in corneal topography measurement,
        139–143, 140f–143f
    and videokeratoscopy, comparison of,
        147–148, 148f
Phakic eye, intraocular lens implanta-
        tion in, 211–216. *See also*
        Intraocular lens implantation,
        in phakic eye
Pharmaceutical agents, myopia control
        with, 129–137
    adrenergic blocking agents,
        133–134, 135t
    apomorphine, future possibilities
        with, 135–136
    atropine, 130–131
    cycloplegic agents, 129–133, 133t
    future possibilities with, 134–136
    labetalol, 134, 135t
    pirenzepine, future possibilities
        with, 135
    timolol, 134, 135t
    tropicamide, 132–133, 133t
Phoria(s)
    dissociated, tests of, 72

effect on reduction of progression
        rates with bifocals, 121–125
    induced, symptoms of myopia due
        to, 66
    tests, associated, in binocular vision
        examination, 73
    vertical, symptoms of myopia due
        to, 66–67
Photoablation, 187
Photo-Electronic keratoscope, 144
Photokeratoscopy, in corneal topogra-
        phy measurement, 144
Photorefractive keratectomy
    comanagement of patients, 201–202
    prevalence of, 203–204
Physiologic myopia, 16
Pirenzepine, myopia control with,
        future possibilities with, 135
Placido's disk, 144
Polymethyl methacrylate lenses,
        myopia control with, 156
Positive fusional vergence reserve, 73
Posterior chamber lenses, in phakic eye,
        214–216, 215t
    complications of, 215–216
    results of studies of, 214–215, 215t
Posterior segment enlargement, 53–54
Posterior staphyloma formation, 33, 34f
Presbyopia
    as factor in prescribing for myopia,
        84, 86
    symptoms of myopia due to, 68
Preschool-aged children, prevalence of
        myopia among, 9–11, 10t
Prescribing for myopia, 77–97
    accommodation considerations in,
        79–84
    accommodative insufficiency in, 81
    age in, 77–78
    basic exophoria in, 83
    case report, 78–79, 82–83, 88–89
    convergence excess in, 80–81
    convergence insufficiency in, 84
    divergence excess in, 83
    general guidelines for, 77–79
    glasses vs. contact lenses, 86–91
    night myopia in, 92–93
    presbyopia in, 84, 86
    pseudoconvergence insufficiency in, 82
    pseudomyopia in, 93–94

vergence considerations in, 79–84
Prevalence, 8–14
  among newborns, 9, 10t
  among preschool-aged children, 9, 10t
  among school-aged children, 9–11, 10t
  in early adult years, 11–12, 11t
  factors related to, 13–14
  graphic representation of, 15, 15f
  in Hong Kong, 14
  in later adult years, 12–13, 12t
  in Singapore, 14
  in Taiwan, 14
Prevention, 58
Prism-neutralized cover test, in binocu-
      lar vision examination, 71–72
Progression, 21–31
  in children, 21–24, 22f, 23t
    ocular optical component changes
      in, 26–28, 27f, 27t
    rates of, 51, 52f
      factors affecting, 24–26, 25t, 26f
  in young adults
    ocular optical component changes
      in, 29–31
    patterns of, 28–29, 28f–30f
Progressive addition lenses, for near
      work, 125
Pseudoconvergence insufficiency, as factor
      in prescribing for myopia, 82
Pseudomyopia, 15
  as factor in prescribing for myopia,
      93–94
  recognition of, 69

Radial keratotomy, 181–187
  anisometropia after, 183
  Casebeer system, 185
  contact lenses after, fitting of, 186
  for correcting astigmatism, 185–186
  ethical issues related to, 186–187
  evaluation of, 182–185
  glare and fluctuating vision after,
      182–183
  historical background of, 181–182
  hyperopic drift after, 184
  innovations in, 185–186
  legal issues related to, 186–187
  loss of best-corrected visual acuity
      after, 183
  mini-radial keratotomy, 185

need for glasses or contact lenses
      after, 183
  predictability of refractive outcome
      with, 183
  traumatic injury after, 184
Refractive error
  heritabilities of, 49–50, 50t
  predictability of, after laser photore-
      fractive keratectomy,
      190–191, 191t
  at school entry, 18
Refractive examination, 68–69
  keratometry in, 68–69
  retinoscopy in, 69
  subjective refraction in, 69
Refractive surgery
  vs. accelerated orthokeratology,
      175–177, 176f
  involving lens, 207–217
    clear lens extraction, 207–217. *See
      also* Clear lens extraction
    intraocular lens implantation in
      phakic eye, 211–216. *See also*
      Intraocular lens implantation,
      in phakic eye
  orthokeratology after, 177–178
Retinal breaks, 36
Retinal detachment, 37–38
  as function of refractive error, proba-
      bility of, 39, 40t
Retinal hemorrhages, 33
Retinal image size, comparison between
      lenses and spectacles, 87
Retinoscopy, in refractive examination, 69
Reverse geometry lenses
  accelerated orthokeratology with,
      167–177
    case reports, 170–172
    fitting Contex OK lenses, 168–170
    Mountford's fitting method, 174
    results with, 170–174
    retrospective and prospective stud-
      ies, 172–174, 173f
  legal status of, 178
Rhegmatogenous retinal detachment, 37
Rigid contact lenses
  control of progression with, 155–163
    gas-permeable, 157–162, 159f,
      160f, 161t
    bifocal lenses, 162–163

Rigid contact lenses – *continued*
  Houston Rigid Gas-Permeable
    Myopia Control Study,
    157–162, 159f, 160f, 161t
  polymethyl methacrylate, 156
  prediction of, 162
  fitting of, videokeratoscopy in, 149–150
  gas-permeable, myopia control with,
    157–162
  orthokeratology with, 163–167
    Berkeley Orthokeratology Study,
      165–166, 166f
    Binder et al. Orthokeratology
      Study, 165
    Houston Orthokeratology Study,
      164–165
    Pacific University Orthokeratology
      Study, 166–167, 168t
  reduction with, 155–180
Risk factors, 16–21, 16t, 17t, 18f, 19t, 20t
  family history, 16, 16t
  refractive error of emmetropia,
    16–19, 17t, 18f

Scanning beam excimer laser, in pho-
    torefractive keratectomy,
    196–197
School-aged children, prevalence of
    myopia among, 9–11, 10t
Scleral crescent, 31
Simple myopia, 15, 16
Singapore, prevalence of myopia in, 14
Spasm of accommodation, symptoms of
    myopia due to, 67
Spectacle(s)
  considerations for, 91–92
  and contact lenses, optical compari-
    son of, 87–88
  part-time wear of, for near work,
    125–126
Staphyloma, posterior, formation of,
    33, 34f
Steep central island, 191
Strabismus, symptoms of myopia due
    to, 67
Subjective cover test, in binocular
    vision examination, 71
Subjective refraction, in refractive
    examination, 69
Subretinal neovascularization, 35

Summit Technology Study, 189, 190t
Symptoms, 63–68
  accommodative insufficiency, 67–68
  anomalies of accommodation, 67
  binocular vision anomalies, 65–68
  esophoria, 66
  exophoria, 66
  fatigue of accommodation, 67
  heterophorias, 65–67
  infacility of accommodation, 67
  paralysis of accommodation, 68
  presbyopia, 68
  pseudomyopia, 67
  spasm of accommodation, 67
  strabismus, 67

Taiwan, prevalence of myopia in, 14
Temporal arc of flashes, 36
Temporal crescent, 31
Timolol, myopia control with, 134, 135t
Tonometry, in ocular health examina-
    tion, 75
Topographic maps, accuracy of,
    145–147, 146f
Topographical Modeling System, 145
Topography, corneal, 139–154. *See also*
    Corneal topography
Transepithelial multipass multizone pho-
    torefractive keratectomy, 197
Transepithelial photorefractive keratec-
    tomy ablation, 197
Traumatic injury, after radial keratot-
    omy, 184
Tropicamide, myopia control with,
    132–133, 133t

Undercorrection, for near work, 125
Unilateral cover test, in binocular
    vision examination, 70

Vergence, as factor in prescribing for
    myopia, 79–84
Vertical phoria, symptoms of myopia
    due to, 66–67
Videokeratoscopy
  in accelerated orthokeratology, 175
  in corneal topography measurement,
    144–153
    accuracy of topographic maps,
      145–147, 146f

applications of, 149–153
  in accelerated orthokeratology
    using reverse geometry
    lenses, 150
  in conventional orthokeratol-
    ogy, 150
  in keratorefractive surgery,
    150–151
  in postoperative monitoring of
    corneal topography, 152–153
  in preoperative screening for
    keratoconus, 151
  in rigid contract lens fitting,
    149–150
  in screening for changes in
    corneal topography due to
    contact lens wear, 151–152
  instruments in, 145, 145t
  and peripheral keratometry, compari-
    son of, 147–148, 148f
Vision
  binocular. *See under* Binocular
    vision
  distance, blurred, 63–65, 64t, 65t
  fluctuating, after radial keratotomy,
    182–183
  in low contrast, after laser photore-
    fractive keratectomy, 194
Vision therapy, 101–111

Baltimore project, 101–102
behavioral training methods studies,
  105–107
biofeedback studies, 102–105
  in myopia control, 107–109
Visual acuity
  best-corrected, loss of
    after laser photorefractive keratec-
      tomy, 191–192
    after radial keratotomy, 183
  distance, myopia and, relationship
    between, 63–64, 64t, 65t
  after laser photorefractive keratec-
    tomy, 190–191, 191t
Visual field screening, in ocular health
  examination, 75
Vitreous detachment, 35–36, 36–37, 37f
von Graefe dissociated phoria test, in
  binocular vision examination,
  70, 72

White-without-pressure, 36

Young adults
  myopia progression in, patterns of,
    28–29, 28f–30f
  prevalence of myopia among,
    11–12, 11t
Youth-onset myopia, 14–15

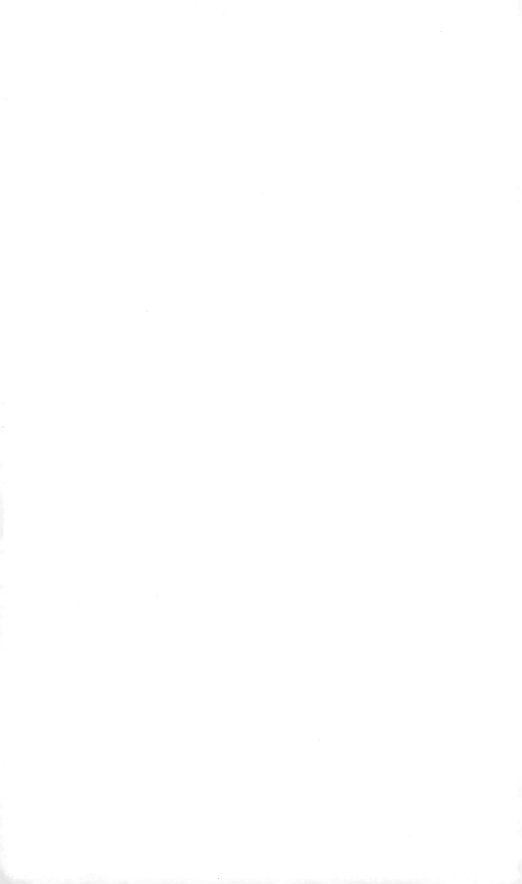